Mariana Policena Rosa
Ida Helena C. F. Menezes
Lucilene Ma. de Sousa

Primary Health Care Quality Assessment

Mariana Policena Rosa
Ida Helena C. F. Menezes
Lucilene Ma. de Sousa

Primary Health Care Quality Assessment

Training and Qualification of Professionals

ScienciaScripts

Imprint

Any brand names and product names mentioned in this book are subject to trademark, brand or patent protection and are trademarks or registered trademarks of their respective holders. The use of brand names, product names, common names, trade names, product descriptions etc. even without a particular marking in this work is in no way to be construed to mean that such names may be regarded as unrestricted in respect of trademark and brand protection legislation and could thus be used by anyone.

Cover image: www.ingimage.com

This book is a translation from the original published under ISBN 978-3-330-77391-2.

Publisher:
Sciencia Scripts
is a trademark of
Dodo Books Indian Ocean Ltd. and OmniScriptum S.R.L publishing group

120 High Road, East Finchley, London, N2 9ED, United Kingdom
Str. Armeneasca 28/1, office 1, Chisinau MD-2012, Republic of Moldova, Europe
Managing Directors: Ieva Konstantinova, Victoria Ursu
info@omniscriptum.com

Printed at: see last page
ISBN: 978-620-3-25927-8

SUMMARY

ACKNOWLEDGMENTS

To Professor Maria do Rosàrio Gondim Peixoto of the Faculty of Nutrition of the Federal University of Goiàs for the statistical support and to the Research Support Foundation of the State of Goiàs for the financial support, call n° 003/ 2013, process n° 201310267000397.

PRESENTATION

The motivation for developing this work comes from the authors' interest and professional work in Collective Health and Health Teaching. These experiences have been developed both in training in Nutrition, a common area between the authors, and in practical work in Collective Health, in the Unified Health System (SUS). As for the subject of the research presented in this book, which deals with the relationship between professional training and qualification and the quality of services provided in Primary Health Care, I became interested in 2012, in the Professional Master's Degree in Health Teaching (MEPES/UFG), in the line of research Educational Processes in Health Work.

The fact that one of the authors works at the Family Health Support Center (NASF) highlights the importance of this professional in providing technical and pedagogical support to the Family Health teams and also as a facilitator in the teaching-learning process and in transforming professional health practices.

In the NASF, the work process is developed through matrix support, with the creation of collective spaces for discussions and planning. There is the organization and structuring of shared care, specific interventions by NASF professionals with users and families and common actions in the territories under their responsibility, including health promotion projects, continuing education for professionals and the organization of the work process of the Family Health teams (BRASIL, 2010a).

In this encounter between teaching, at MEPES, and service, at NASF, the authors identify the need to analyze factors related to the training and qualification of Family Health Strategy professionals associated with the quality of Primary Care services.

We believe that the content of this book will be of interest to teachers and academics in the health field, managers and workers of the SUS and actors of social control and will contribute to the reorientation of teaching and services, to the qualification of educational processes in health work, and consequently, to the quality of health and life of the population, positively impacting the communities served, the great purpose of health work.

The book is organized into nine chapters. The Introduction (Chapter 1) contextualizes the topic, the concepts that permeate it and their importance, the problem, guiding question, justification and main objective of the study.

Chapters 2 to 5 explore, in the light of the literature, the historical process, concepts, main studies and the importance of the training and qualification of professionals to work in the health area, especially in Primary Health Care (PHC) and evaluation of its quality, as well as the relationship between the training and qualification profile of professionals and the quality of PHC.

The study's methodological approach is described in Chapter 6. In this chapter, the reader can learn about the type, location and population of the study, the data collection process and instruments used, the study variables, data analysis and the ethical aspects of the research.

Chapter 7 describes the training profile, professional experience and qualifications of the professionals interviewed, the presence and extent of PHC attributes in the services evaluated and the relationship between the training profile and qualifications of the professionals and the quality of PHC services.

Chapter 8 answers whether factors related to professional training and qualification influence the quality of PHC and how this relationship occurs, and finally, chapter 9 presents the conclusion of the study.

It should be noted that this book is a product of the dissertation submitted to the Postgraduate Program in Health Teaching at the Professional Master's level of the Federal University of Goiás for defense purposes and the article published in the Brazilian Journal of Medical Education, entitled "Training and qualification of health professionals: factors associated with the quality of Primary Care" (OLIVEIRA *et al.*, 2016).

The study was partially presented as a poster at the Research, Teaching and Extension Congress (CONPEEX/UFG) in 2013, delivered as a Technical Report to the Goiânia Municipal Health Department in 2014 and used in the diagnosis and planning of the Family Health teams during the Primary Care Planning in 2016 (BRASIL, 2011a).

CHAPTER 1

INTRODUCTION

Health education for the training and qualification of professionals is a historical process that has been updated over time (COSTA, 2006).

In this trajectory, the twentieth century was marked by legal frameworks and movements for changes in the training of health professionals, with the aim of overcoming the models of higher education in health that are still tied to a model of hospital-centered and fragmented practice, with a privatizing bias, and are deficient in meeting the social needs for health, presenting little or no relationship with the social and epidemiological reality of the population (BRASIL, 2007a).

Although these movements did not achieve all of their objectives, progress was made in the direction of teaching and care that was more appropriate to the reality of society, from the perspective of quality Primary Health Care (PHC) (GONZALEZ; ALMEIDA, 2010).

Similarly, in the field of the qualification of professionals working in the Unified Health System (SUS), concern about the education of health professionals has been endorsed by social movements, legislation and public policies which argue that a health system should require a reorientation of policies for managing work and education in health, defining guidelines for the sector and strengthening the integration of teaching, service and community (CONFERÊNCIA NACIONAL DE SAÙDE, 8ª, 1987).

In this sense, Permanent Education in Health (EPS) was defended as a fundamental strategy for reorganizing training, care, management, policy-making and social control practices in the health sector, through intersectoral actions and changes in health teaching, thus constituting a quadrilateral made up of different actors in the work process: care, teaching, management and social control (CECCIM; FEURWERKER, 2004; COSTA, 2006; CECCIM;

FERLA, 2008).

PHC is a way of organizing health services, a strategy for integrating all aspects of these services, with the population's health needs in mind (BRASIL, 2011b).

The concept of PHC and its principles were consolidated in the 20th century, which was marked by the development of various experiments in health care models around the world. These experiences served as the basis for establishing the principles of PHC proposed in the Alma Ata Declaration in 1978. From then on, the strengthening of PHC was established as the main strategy for organizing public health services (LEÂO; CALDEIRA; OLIVEIRA, 2011).

In Brazil, the Family Health Strategy (ESF) is considered the main strand of PHC and aims to implement and strengthen the SUS, proposing to reorganize the practice of health care on new bases and replace the traditional model, bringing health closer to families and thereby improving the quality of life of the population (BRASIL, 2010a).

PHC is defined by its attributes, which are recognized worldwide as the structuring axes of the care process, associated with the quality of services and the effectiveness and efficiency of its interventions: first contact access to the SUS, the

longitudinality, comprehensive care, coordination of care, family and community orientation and cultural competence (STARFIELD, 2002; ZILS et al., 2009).

Training and qualification in PHC are associated with the quest to guarantee the universality and comprehensiveness of the SUS, since, in addition to comprising an assigned territory based on a family and community approach, PHC is considered a space for collective construction, where different subjects are involved in health care (D'AVILA, 2014).

The studies by Kolling (2008); Castro (2012); Chomatas; Vitória (2013), who assessed the quality of PHC services through its attributes in the perception of doctors and nurses in cities in the southern region of Brazil, using the Primary Care Assessment Tool (PCATool) (BRASIL, 2010b), reveal that a better result in terms of PHC attributes is related, among other factors, to better training and qualification of its professionals. However, even after advances in PHC policies and practices in Brazil in recent years, there are obstacles to their consolidation, both socio-political and structural, as well as those related to the work process (FIGUEIREDO, 2011; NASCIMENTO, 2011).

In Goiânia, the Municipal Health Department (SMS) has been implementing actions under the National Policy for Permanent Education in Health (PNEPS), which is currently coordinated by the Municipal School of Public Health, of the Directorate for Work Management and Education in Health.

The PNEPS, established by Ministerial Order No 198 of February 2004, states that the management of health education, through the training and development of health workers, is a fundamental issue for the quality of health care provided to the population and a strategy for qualifying the management of health services and systems (BRASIL, 2004a).

The work of one of the authors in the northwestern region at the Family Health Support Center (NASF) led the authors to question the effective contribution of academic training and professional qualification courses and training on the practices and concepts of Primary Health Care, which are still very fragmented and from an outpatient, biomedical perspective, and their impact on the quality of the services provided to the population.

The north-western region was chosen for this study because it is the *site of* pilot projects in continuing education, the health district with the highest FHS coverage in the municipality (51%) and the only one currently with an NASF.

Training and events are held every year, as well as partnerships in postgraduate courses, in order to disseminate knowledge and qualify health professionals to work in PHC. However, there are no records of studies that have analyzed the effectiveness of training and qualification strategies for professionals in relation to the quality of PHC services in the municipality.

According to Castro (2012), who studied the profile of medical and nursing professionals in Porto Alegre associated with the quality of PHC services, knowledge of the profile of professionals in terms of academic training, continuing education and occupational characteristics, associated with the quality of these services, is fundamental for promoting improvements in both the training and qualification of health professionals to work in PHC.

Given this context, and relating it to the professional practice of one of the authors in the NASF, in which she works directly in matrix support and continuing education for the Family Health teams, this study poses the following guiding question: what factors related to the qualification and training of health professionals are associated with the quality of services in the northwestern region of Goiânia?

This study aims to analyze the factors related to the training and qualification of Family Health Strategy professionals associated with the quality of Primary Care services.

CHAPTER 2

TRAINING THE HEALTH PROFESSIONAL

Education is understood not only as an institutional and instructional process, but also as a formative instrument, whether in the particularity of the personal pedagogical relationship, or in the context of the collective social relationship without losing ethical and political references, with the premise that the process of forming an ethical subject, or a citizen, will depend on the construction of the human being itself (CECCiM; FERLA, 2008).

The 20th century was marked by intense scientific progress and the devaluation of empiricism in health care. Proposed by Abraham Flexner, an American doctor, in the 1910s, the so-called Flexner Report consolidated the paradigm of scientific medicine, which guided, and still guides in many places, teaching and professional practices in the health sector throughout the 20th century. Its main characteristics are: the segmentation of teaching into basic and professional cycles, teaching based on disciplines or specialties and mostly set within hospitals, with a fragmented vision and reduced to the biological aspects of health (GONZALEZ; ALMEIDA, 2010).

In Brazil, the flexinerian model arrived in the 1940s, influencing new courses in medicine, dentistry and nursing, as well as reformulating existing courses. University education was formed in such a way as to separate objects from their contexts, dividing content into disciplines that do not integrate and are incapable of understanding the complexity of reality. In this model, health care is centered on curative, hospital and super-specialized care, in line with economic and corporate interests (GoNZALEZ; ALMEIDA, 2010).

However, the growing expenditure on investments in technology, the unbridled consumption of diagnostic and treatment possibilities in contrast to the scarcity of resources to pay for them are key points in the downfall of this model, especially in poor or developing countries. Even so, the paradigms of the

Flexinerian model have become so ingrained in health teaching and practice that they predominate today. Replacing this system with the universal system, which seeks care models that value comprehensiveness, humanized care and health promotion, depends on the training profile and practice of health professionals (GONZALEZ; ALMEIDA, 2010).

The discussion about a broader concept of health, beyond the biological aspects, stimulated a rethink in several European and American countries about the issue of health care and teaching. The proposal for preventive reform and comprehensive medicine emerged, encompassing health in the health-disease process (GONZALEZ; ALMEIDA, 2010).

In Brazil, in the 1950s, two major movements for change in the higher education of health professionals emerged: Community Medicine, which sought to revive medicine prior to the great technological explosion, with differentiated inclusion of marginalized social strata and encouragement of community participation, especially voluntary work, and the Integration of Teaching and Care (IDA), instituted by the Ministry of Education, which sought to break down students' resistance to the epidemiological and social approach, inserting them into primary care through outreach activities, which happened intensively in the 1970s (DIAS et al., 2013).

These movements emerged with the aim of responding to the limitations of access to the service system due to excessive spending on technology. However, these strategies did not change hospital-centered teaching and fragmented practice in numerous specialties. IDA was limited to health care, with low teacher participation and segmentation of actions, not resulting in significant transformations in curricula. Although the final goal of these movements was not achieved, much progress has been made towards teaching and care that is more appropriate to the reality of society (DIAS et al., 2013; GONZALEZ; ALMEIDA, 2010).

The Alma-Ata meeting in 1978, held on the occasion of the International

Conference on Primary Health Care, resulted in reformist advances, mainly the PHC strategy, and led to strong reforms in several countries, strengthening the Health Reform movement in Brazil. After Alma-Ata, discussions began on how to insert university work into the health service and the idea was reached that the service precedes the university and the university should not intend to structure it (GONZALEZ; ALMEIDA, 2010).

The shock at the rising costs of health care, the insufficiency and dehumanization of health care made the need for a change in training and the effective participation of the community in drawing up and monitoring the process even more evident (GONZALEZ; ALMEIDA, 2010).

These movements led the *Kellogg* Foundation to start the UNI Program (A New Initiative in the Training of Health Professionals: Union with the Community) in 1993 in the municipality of Botucatu/SP, which brought together three movements: IDA, APS and Community Outreach. Based on cooperation and shared management between the university, local health services and community organizations, this program aimed to guide health training from the perspective of multiprofessionalism, strengthen internships in the community, rethink the university, make it relevant to society and stimulate academic production with social participation (DIAS et al., 2013; GONZALEZ; ALMEIDA, 2010; KISIL M.; CHAVES M., 1994; MACHADO, J. L. M.; CALDAS JR, A. L.; BORTONCELLO, N. M. F., 1997).

Through this initiative, UNI contributed to a new way of integrating partners and developing models, paving the way for the training of health professionals who could articulate scientific and technological advances to the needs of the population and intensified the union between the three major components and actors of the pro-change movement: university, service and community. There was thus a breakthrough in these movements, with interdisciplinary learning at university and multi-professionalism in services and the community being valued (DIAS et al., 2013; GONZALEZ; ALMEIDA, 2010; KISIL M.; CHAVES

M., 1994; MACHADO, J. L. M.; CALDAS JR, A. L.; BORTONCELLO, N. M. F., 1997).

The university's effective participation in these projects triggered a new movement in 1997, the Rede Unida (United Network), which brought together actors and institutions around changes and new experiences for professional health training, with the great challenge of preventing the continuation of fragmentation and including integrality and humanization in practices while still in training (DIAS et al., 2013; GONZALEZ; DE ALMEIDA, 2010).

In a survey on the profile of medical schools carried out by the National Interinstitutional Commission for the Evaluation of Medical Schools (CINAEM) in 1991, the results showed the inadequacy of medical training in relation to the demands of society and confirmed the presence of the hegemonic paradigm of teacher-centered teaching, overspecialization and actions aimed at the tertiary sector (GONZALEZ; ALMEIDA, 2010).

The excessive specialization observed in the health sector has been pointed out, among other factors, as one of the reasons for the rise in healthcare costs and the poor geographical distribution of professionals in this area. This is not to deny the importance of specialization, but it is essential to seek a balance in the ratio of specialists to generalists, without jeopardizing the quality of care provided. In general, specialization is reinforced by the development of scientific research, which predominantly focuses on high-tech aspects (BRASIL, 2007a).

In parallel to the CINAEM movement, other studies promoted by the IDA project concluded that the teaching-service articulation strategy should be rethought in order to involve multi-professional teams throughout the undergraduate course and that the limited participation of the community should be stimulated so that it takes place in a conscious and co-responsible manner (GONZALEZ; ALMEIDA, 2010).

Among the challenges facing the SUS and the University in training health workers, new models are needed that are technologically competent, encourage teamwork, are creative, autonomous, problem-solving, engaged in health promotion, open to social participation and committed to humanizing health care (ALMEIDA FILHO, 2013).

In this sense, the Law of Guidelines and Bases of National Education No. 9.394, of December 20, 1996 (BRASIL, 1996), gives Higher Education Institutions (HEIs) new degrees of freedom that make it possible to design innovative curricula, suited to regional realities and the respective vocations of the schools. The replacement of the minimum curriculum by the National Curriculum Guidelines for undergraduate health courses (DCNs) represents a step forward, as it induces greater articulation between HEIs (BRASIL, 2007a).

The DCNs were approved by the National Health Council between 2001 and 2002, but each profession had its guidelines published separately, and they were approved for the 14 health courses between 2001 and 2004. They sought to build an academic and professional profile with competencies, skills and content in line with the current needs of the population, as well as to act with quality and resolution in the SUS (GONZALEZ; ALMEIDA, 2010).

The DCNs for health training include an advanced idea of curriculum formatting. The DCNs advocate articulation between higher education and the health system, general and specific training, with competences common to all professional training, emphasis on health concepts, health promotion, SUS principles and guidelines, teaching-learning with ample freedom of curricular integration, academic and professional profile, competences, skills and contemporary content, capacity to act with quality and resolution in the SUS (ALMEIDA FILHO, 2013; BRASIL, 2001).

Shortly after the approval of the DCNs for medical courses, the Program to Encourage Curricular Changes in Medical Courses (PROMED) was established in 2002 by the Ministry of Health (MS), the Ministry of Education (MEC) and the Pan American Health Organization (PAHO), in partnership with the Brazilian Association of Medical Education (ABEM) and Rede Unida (BRAZIL, 2002). PROMED encouraged the implementation and consolidation of the necessary changes in medical training, encouraging the offer of curricular internships in university hospitals and primary care services, seeking to meet the needs of society and the health sector in accordance with the DCNs and the SUS (DIAS et al., 2013; GONZALEZ; ALMEIDA, 2010).

The creation of the Department of Health Education (DEGES) in 2003 showed that the Ministry of Health was prioritizing changes in higher education. DEGES had the task of motivating and proposing actions both for changes in technical, undergraduate and postgraduate training and for the continuing education of health workers based on the health needs of the population and the strengthening of the SUS (ALMEIDA FILHO, 2013; BRASIL, 2001; DIAS et al., 2013).

Through DEGES, the Ministry of Health and the Ministry of Education have developed various programs to structure and strengthen the process of training and developing human resources in the health area, such as (DIAS et al., 2013; GONZALEZ; ALMEIDA, 2010):

VERSUS (Vivência-Estâgio na Realidade do SUS), instituted between 2003 and 2004, whose design recognized the SUS as a learning space, strengthening relations between training institutions and the health system.

Aprender SUS (Learning SUS), launched in 2004, played an important role in the debate on the integrality of care as an axis of change in professional training, seeking to strengthen cooperation between the health system and higher education institutions (BRASIL, 2004b; DIAS et al., 2013).

The Specialization Course in Activating Processes of Change in the Health Professions, conceptually oriented by the integrated curriculum, constructivism and active and distance learning teaching methodologies, aimed to support the management of teaching in coherence with the constitutional guidelines and principles of the SUS and the implementation of the national curriculum guidelines for undergraduate courses in the health area (BRASIL, 2004b; DIAS et al., 2013).

The National Program for the Reorientation of Professional Training in Health (PRÓ-Saùde), strongly based on PROMED and instituted by Interministerial Ordinance MS/MEC No. 2,101 of November 3, 2005 (BRASIL, 2005). Initially designed for the areas of Nursing, Medicine and Dentistry, it was later extended to other undergraduate courses in the Health area through Interministerial Ordinance MS/MEC no. 3.019, of November 27, 2007, aims to integrate teaching and service, with a view to reorienting professional training, ensuring a comprehensive approach to the health-disease process with an emphasis on primary care, promoting transformations in the processes of generating knowledge, teaching and learning and providing services to the population (BRASIL, 2007a).

The Education through Work for Health Program (PET- Saùde), established by Interministerial Ordinance MS/MEC No. 421 of March 3, 2010, which promotes the formation of tutorial learning groups for development of activities in strategic areas of the SUS. It encourages teaching-service-community integration through the insertion of teachers and undergraduate students in the public health network, so that the needs of the services are a source of knowledge production and research in educational institutions. It develops projects in the areas of FHS, Health Surveillance and Mental Health (BRASIL, 2010c).

Despite advances in the concepts and programs of higher education in health in Brazil, the predominant orientation in training is still alien to the sectoral organization and the critical debate on health care, with little relation to the social and epidemiological reality of the population (BRASIL, 2007a).

Higher education models in health are still tied to a hospital-centric and fragmented model of practice, with a privatizing bias, and are proving to be deficient in meeting the social needs for health. The predominant profile of graduates from health courses reveals their lack of commitment to the SUS and understanding of the need for teamwork, poor humanistic training, often resulting in unprepared professionals (ALMEIDA FILHO, 2013).

In this regime, which is still hegemonic in Brazilian universities, curricula are more closed, designed for exclusivity in training, and tend to be less interdisciplinary and more specialized, thus alienating professional segments from each other and hindering efficient teamwork. There is almost no room for more general studies, which are necessary to promote a broad humanistic view of diseases and health care by health professionals, within the critical framework of the Social Determination of Health (ALMEIDA FILHO, 2013; BRASIL, 2007a).

As for the pedagogical approach, it is often limited to traditional methodologies based on the transmission of knowledge, which do not favor the critical formation of the student, inserting them late in the world of work. The interdisciplinary approach and working in multi-professional teams are rarely explored by undergraduate training institutions, which is reproduced in health teams, resulting in the isolated action of each professional and the overlapping of care actions and their fragmentation (BRASIL, 2007a).

CHAPTER 3

HEALTH PROFESSIONAL QUALIFICATION

Educational approaches to the training and qualification of health professionals have undergone profound changes and updates over time (BRASIL, 2009a; COSTA, 2006).

In this evolution, educating for health work should no longer be about transferring cognitive and technological resources to new generations of professionals, but about training people who are committed to implementing a project for society, where health is largely related to quality of life and work (CECCIM; FERLA, 2008).

On the other hand, these transformations in educational processes seek to consolidate the Brazilian Health Reform, by strengthening the decentralization of sector management, developing strategies and processes to achieve comprehensive individual and collective health care and increasing society's participation in SUS policy decisions (BRASIL, 2007b).

In this sense, the concern with the education of health professionals has been referenced since the III National Health Conference (CNS) in 1963, still with a vision focused on training, technical improvement and specialization of health work (COSTA, 2006).

The CNSs that took place between the 1960s and 1980s brought new elements to health education, such as the importance of the health professional as a resource that should be developed to promote progress and social well-being and continuing education as a dynamic teaching-learning process, active and permanent, aimed at updating and improving people's capacity in the face of scientific and technological development (COSTA, 2006). In this historical process, some concepts of health education have emerged.

In the 1960s and 1970s, the most widely used concept was in-service education, which was a set of educational practices designed to help workers act more effectively in order to directly achieve the institution's objectives. It was the first concept put into practice by the CNSs, as a way of adjusting professionals to the health needs of public services (COSTA, 2006; FARAH, 2003; OLIVEIRA et al., 2011).

In the 1980s, the concept of "continuing education" emerged, which was defined as a set of continuing educational practices subsequent to initial training, which allow workers to maintain, increase or improve their competence, so that it is compatible with the development of their responsibilities, thus characterizing competence as an individual attribute, aimed at developing potential, for a change in attitudes and behaviors in the cognitive, affective and psychomotor areas of the human being, with a view to transforming their practice (COSTA, 2006; OLIVEIRA et al., 2011).

In Brazil, the concept of Permanent Education in Health (EPS) is the result of reflection on the process of training and development of health professionals and the unfolding of movements for change in health care, with a view to improving the quality of services and adapting them to the real health needs of the population (COSTA, 2006).

For the MoH, EPS is understood as:

"a proposal for strategic action capable of contributing to the transformation of training processes, pedagogical and health practices and the organization of services, undertaking a joint effort between the health system, in its various spheres of management, and training institutions" (Brazil, 2004a, p.9).

From the 1980s onwards, PHE was taken on as a priority by PAHO and the World Health Organization (WHO), which guided the countries of the American continent through guidelines, programs and some policies in the area of human resources development (FERRAZ, 2012).

Among the Health Reform movements, the 8th CNS, in March 1986, argued that a National Health System should require a reorientation of labor management and health education policies, with the definition of policies for the sector and the strengthening of teaching-service integration. This meant rethinking the traditional proposals for integrating teaching and care (CONFERÊNCIA NACIONAL DE SAÙDE, 8ª, 1987).

In the Federal Constitution of 1988, through Article 200, III (BRASIL, 1988) and Law No. 8080, of September 19, 1990 (BRASIL, 1990), the SUS assumes the competence to organize training in the health area (BRASIL, 2009a; 2009b).

From this normatization, in Brazil, the EPS gained prominence within the health system with the VIII CNS and the I and II National Conferences on Human Resources (1986 and 1993). The events and discussions that have taken place over the last few decades served as the basis for drawing up the Basic Operational Standard for Human Resources in Health (NOB/HR/SUS) proposed in 1996 and approved in 2002 (BRASIL, 2003; COSTA, 2006; FERRAZ, 2012).

The NOB/HR/SUS proposed actions and norms for a greater commitment from the three spheres of government to implement an EPS model focused on the attributions and competencies of SUS workers (FERRAZ, 2012).

With Ministerial Ordinance 198 of February 13, 2004 (BRASIL, 2004a), the Ministry of Health established the PNEPS with the aim of transforming and qualifying the practices of training, care, management, social control and popular participation; the organization of health services and their respective work processes; the pedagogical practices of training and development of health workers (BRASIL, 2004c; BRASIL, 2009a; CECCIM, 2005).

To strengthen the PNEPS, the Ministry of Health issued Ordinance No. 1996 of August 20, 2007 (BRASIL, 2007b; BRASIL, 2009a), which defines the guidelines for implementing the EPS as a national policy for the training and development of health workers, with a view to linking the possibilities of developing the education of professionals with the expansion of the resolution capacity of health services. This public policy proposes that worker training processes take as a reference the health needs of people and populations, sector management and social control in health (PEDUZZI et al., 2009).

The strengthening of the PNEPS is also advocated within PHC, by the National Primary Care Policy (PNAB) (BRASIL, 2006; BRASIL, 2011c), which defines as common responsibilities for all SUS managers to agree and allocate budgetary and financial resources to strengthen the PNEPS and implement the guidelines for training and continuing education in line with local or regional realities (BRASIL, 2011b).

The PNEPS, in making explicit the proposal's relationship with the principles and guidelines of the SUS, proposes breaking with the concept of a vertical system to work with the idea of a network, in an articulated set of basic, specialized and hospital services in which all health actions and services are provided, recognizing contexts and life histories and ensuring adequate reception and accountability for the health problems of people and populations, considering that practices are defined by multiple factors (BRASIL, 2009a).

EPS is based on the concept of education as transformation and meaningful learning, through problematizing the worker's reality, in the context of their experiences, encouraging changes in educational strategies with contextualized and participatory forms of teaching, in order to focus on practice as a source of knowledge and get the professional actively involved in the educational process (BRASIL, 2009a; BRASIL, 2011b; JESUS et al, 2011; PEDUZZI et al., 2009; TESSER et al., 2011).

Thus, EPS is a fundamental public policy for transforming work in the sector so that it becomes a place for critical, reflective, committed and technically competent action. Currently, continuing education has been considered an important tool in building professional competence, contributing to the organization of work (CECCIM, 2005; OLIVEIRA et al., 2011).

Furthermore, EPS is a fundamental strategy for reorganizing training, care, management, policy-making and social control practices in the health sector, through intersectoral actions and changes in health teaching, thus forming a quadrilateral made up of different actors in the work process: care, teaching, management and social control (CECCIM; FERLA, 2008; CECCIM; FEURWERKER, 2004; COSTA, 2006).

According to Tesser (2011), EPS is a privileged instrument for analyzing reality and building health promotion and care actions in the ESF and overcoming the hierarchical and authoritarian view of education and work processes, qualifying the training and practices of PHC health professionals.

Despite the progress made in PHC policies and practices in Brazil, it has its limits, presenting obstacles to its consolidation, both socio-political and structural, as well as those related to the work process (BRASIL, 2011b; FIGUEIREDO, 2011; NASCIMENTO, 2011).

These obstacles are rooted in the process of training professionals, which, despite efforts to change it, is still far removed from the needs of the SUS, especially the ESF (BRASIL, 2011b). Traditional health training, based on disciplinary organization and specialties, leads to the fragmented study of people's and societies' health problems, leading to the training of specialists who are unable to deal with totalities or complex realities, such as those found in the ESF (CARDOSO et al., 2005).

The central obstacle, from which many others derive, is the lack of political and social valorization of PHC, which faces many challenges in becoming hegemonic as a proposal capable of confronting the existing fragmented model. Another difficulty is the inclusion of new professionals in the PHC proposal, since most of those working in the system are still trained in a privatized care model (BRASIL, 2011b).

Another obstacle to the consolidation of PHC is related to human resources and the training and continuing education of professionals and managers, which often do not include aspects of PHC, from the perspective of meeting social demand, of a resolutive and efficient health system (BRASIL, 2011b).

In general, the training model that predominates among us trains technicians who are competent but not very committed to public health policies, lacking a critical view of society and health, with an attitude that is not very humanistic and far removed from the values of health promotion. Professionals with such training are generally resistant to change and tend to defend the *status quo*, distanced from critical knowledge of the political, social and cultural aspects that structure the theoretical framework of the Social Determination of Health (ALMEIDA FILHO, 2011).

In this context, it is the role of the public sector, in its process of planning and executing health actions, to make available, through continuing education and EPS, the development of skills for the adoption of soft technologies, recognizing the importance of continuity of care, the professional/service-user relationship and the team's ability to understand their role as resource managers, which will be fundamental in the final result (BRASIL, 2011b).

Thus, there is a need to promote a more humanistic, critical-social and generalist qualification of health professionals to work in PHC, through EPS, which works with tools that seek critical reflection on the daily practice of health services and enables changes in the work process, either through training promoted by the service or courses and postgraduate courses in Collective Health, with an emphasis on PHC (BRASIL, 2009a; BRASIL, 2011b; LUZ, 2010).

The social recognition of these professionals, adequate remuneration, the adoption of career plans, the guarantee of labor and social security rights, the improvement of the infrastructure of the units, the possibility of qualification, enabling the training and permanent education of the teams and stimulating intellectual production are crucial for the retention of professionals and the viability of the principles of PHC (BRASIL, 2011b; BRASIL, 2011c).

CHAPTER 4

PRIMARY HEALTH CARE

Alongside the changes that took place in education, the 20th century was marked by many transformations in health concepts and practices in Brazil and around the world. The Cartesian and fragmented view of the human being that had been disseminated for centuries, combined with the rise of capitalism and technological development, with a significant increase in social inequalities and political, economic and demographic changes, culminated in health models centered on disease and excluding significant portions of the population (PAIM et al., 2011; RIBEIRO, 2007).

With a hospital-centric and specialized practice, with a privatizing bias, associated with great social disparities, health care was predominantly curative, proving incapable of meeting social needs for health (ALMEIDA FILHO, 2011).

The recognition of these situations led Britain in 1920 to publish the Dawson Report, a PHC project that presented an organizational structure based on different levels of care, the most basic being the primary health care center (STARFIELD, 2002).

Between 1950 and 1970, the WHO searched for experiences of health care models around the world and directed its technical support towards strengthening basic health services, publicizing and promoting regional conferences (1977-1978) that culminated in the formulation of the strategic principles of PHC (ALMEIDA FILHO, 2013).

The Alma Ata Declaration (ORGANIZACIÓN MUNDIAL DE LA SALUD, 1978) reaffirmed the importance of PHC as a principle for all the world's health systems (STARFIELD, 2002). In this, PHC was defined as:

"essential health care based on practical, scientifically well-founded and socially acceptable methods and technologies, made available to all individuals and families in the community, through their full participation, and at a cost that the community and the country can afford at each stage of its development, in the spirit of self-confidence and self-determination. They are an integral part of the country's health system and represent the first level of contact between the individual, the family and the community and the national health system. They should be brought as close as possible to the places where people live and work, and constitute the first element of a continuous process of health care" (ORGANIZACIÓN MUNDIAL DE LA SALUD, 1978, Article VI).

The strengthening of PHC was established at Alma Ata as the main strategy for organizing public health services, with the aim of improving the capacity of health systems to respond to the needs of the population, as opposed to the model centred on specialist doctors and hospitals (BRASIL, 2011b; LEÂO; CALDEIRA; OLIVEIRA, 2011).

Over the years, different interpretations of the breadth and scope of primary care in different countries and continents, its conceptual complexity and the evolution of its implementation have led to derivations that indicate progress or specificity in relation to the original proposal and the use of different terms to name this form of organization of health service systems (BRASIL, 2011 b).

In Brazil, PHC is in line with the SUS guidelines and aims for a health system that emphasizes social equity, co-responsibility between the population and the public sector, solidarity, based on a broad concept of health, being the main gateway to the health system and the place responsible for organizing health care for individuals, their families and the population over time (BRASIL, 2011b).

Different interpretations of PHC are also presented in the Brazilian historical process. The notion that "primary health care, by assuming, in the first half of the 1980s, the character of a simplified medicine program for the poor, rather than a strategy of reorientation of the health services system", led the Ministry of Health to adopt the nomenclature of Primary Care to differentiate it from PHC (CASRO, 2009; GIL, 2006). to differentiate it from PHC (CASTRO, 2009; GIL, 2006).

Although the term "Atençâo Bàsica" is widely used in the country, the Department of Primary Health Care of the Ministry of Health currently considers that both terms have very similar meanings. However, the terminology Atençâo Primària à Saù better represents the proposal of the ESF, and being an internationally defined and established term, it facilitates translations into other languages, adding value to Brazilian and/or Portuguese publications and for these reasons it will be adopted in this study (CASTRO, 2009).

Currently, the concept of PHC that has been used in Brazil, through the ESF, places the country at the forefront of the discussion in the world, as it proposes a strategy for reorienting the care model, with the family as the focus of approach, a defined territory, client adscription, interdisciplinary teamwork, co-responsibility, comprehensiveness, resolutiveness and intersectoriality as its principles (BRASIL, 2011b).

However, even considering an expanded, comprehensive and inclusive Primary Care, in some places we can see focused or exclusionary PHC taking place, where we can observe a huge range of practices under the designation of Primary Care or Family Health (BRASIL, 2011 b).

Evidence shows that PHC has the capacity to respond to 85% of the population's health needs, by providing preventive, curative, rehabilitative and health promotion services; integrating care when there is more than one problem; dealing with the context of life; and influencing people's responses to their health problems (BRASIL, 2011b).

In Brazil, the ESF is considered to be the main strand and organizational strategy of PHC (BRASIL, 2011c). In parallel with the increase in its coverage, there is a growing association between better health outcomes and greater presence and extension of PHC attributes.

The Family Health Survey in Brazil, based on the evolution of health indicators from 1998 to 2004, showed that the FHS is a factor in generating social equity, with a reduction in indicators related to morbidity and mortality (BRASIL, 2006).

Studies by Macinko, Guanais and Souza; Roncalli and Lima (2006); Macinho et al. (2007) and Aquino, Oliveira and Barreto (2009), in all regions of the country, between 1990 and 2004, indicated that the increase in FHS coverage was related to a reduction in infant mortality, to varying but significant degrees.

PHC has thus become one of the most equitable and efficient ways of organizing a health system. In view of the advances made by PHC, it is important to evaluate the results achieved in terms of the organization and supply of services, as well as the possible impact on the population's health (HAUSER et al., 2013).

CHAPTER 5

EVALUATING THE QUALITY OF PRIMARY HEALTH CARE

One of the main references in the evaluation of health services, Donabedian (1990), proposed that the quality of a service can be measured, and therefore evaluated, through three axes, which are closely interlinked - structure, process and result - and demonstrates that an adequate structure is essential in order to achieve satisfactory care processes and, consequently, health results.

Different conceptual models have been developed to evaluate the quality of health care, many starting with Donabedian and also including PHC attributes. The growing interest in evaluating and improving management, planning and quality in health care has stimulated the development of a large number of tools to evaluate health services from the perspective of users, health professionals and managers (FIGUEIREDO, 2011 ; HAUSER et al., 2013).

PHC has unique aspects that characterize it and differentiate it from other levels of care. Starfield (2002), based on Donabedian's framework, proposes a conceptual model for measuring the quality of services provided to a person or population in PHC, based on four essential attributes (first contact access, longitudinality, comprehensiveness and coordination of care) and three derived attributes (family orientation, community orientation and cultural competence).

First contact access addresses the role of PHC as the gateway to the health system, except in emergency situations. It means access to and use of the health service for each new health event or new episode of the same event, being the first resource to be sought when there is a health need/problem (BRASIL, 2011b; CASTRO, 2009; OLIVEIRA et al., 2013).

longitudinality or *continuous* care *is* a relationship of bonding and responsibility that is established over time between individuals and a health professional or team, enabling the monitoring of the various moments in the life cycle of individuals, their families and the community itself, as a regular source of care

(BRASIL, 2011c; CASTRO, 2009; OLIVEIRA et al., 2013).

Comprehensive care or *integrality is* the ability of the health team to deal with the wide range of health needs of the individual, family or communities, either by resolving them, or by making arrangements so that they can receive any type of attention required, whether or not perceived by people (BRASIL, 2011c; CASTRO, 2009; OLIVEIRA et al., 2013).

The *coordination of care*, the essence of which is information, is fundamental to the success of the other attributes, as it allows the various needs of individuals, their families and communities to be identified and a multidisciplinary team to take action to respond to these needs, coordinating actions and responses (BRASIL, 2011c; OLIVEIRA et al., 2013).

With regard to the attributes derived from PHC, *family orientation* or *family focus* addresses the extent to which PHC concentrates on the health of individuals in the context of the family, considering their potential for care and also health threats, including the use of family approach tools. *Community orientation* recognizes the health needs of the community through direct contact and epidemiological data, promoting joint planning and evaluation of services. Finally, *cultural competence* deals with relationships with people from different groups and cultures, seeking to value the cultural characteristics, beliefs and values of the population in the relationship and communication between professionals and the community (BRASIL, 2010b; OLIVEIRA et al., 2013).

Operationalizing the concept of PHC in terms of attributes makes it possible to identify the degree of orientation towards PHC, which makes it possible to compare systems or types of services, as well as the association between the presence of attributes and the effectiveness of care, both at an individual and population level (HARZHEIM et al., 2013).

From this perspective, Barbara Starfield and collaborators at *Johns Hopkins University*, between 1997 and 2001, developed the *Primary Care Assessment*

Tool (PCATool), a set of primary care assessment instruments that measures the extent of PHC attributes by analyzing aspects of structure and process. The PCATool is presented in two versions aimed at children and adult users and a third aimed at health professionals (CHOMATAS, et al., 2013).

In the instrument, some attributes are made up of more than one component, with several items. For example, the completeness attribute is made up of the 'services available' component and the 'services provided' component (HAUSER et al., 2013).

The PCATool has been translated and adapted in several countries with different health systems, including Brazil, Spain, Canada, South Korea, Hong Kong and Argentina (HAUSER et al., 2013).

In Brazil, in particular, two different adaptations of the PCATool, called the Primary Care Assessment Instrument, have been carried out, as well as different processes for assessing validity and reliability. The adaptation carried out by Harzheim et al. (2013), at the PHC Research Group of the Postgraduate Program in Epidemiology at the Rio Grande do Sul School of Medicine, was applied in Porto Alegre, maintaining the original format of the instrument and assessing the validity and reliability of the child and adult user versions. On the other hand, an adaptation carried out by Almeida and Macinko (2006) was used in Petrópolis, Rio de Janeiro, and resulted in the validation of the child user, adult user and health professional versions (HAUSER et al., 2013).

For health professionals, it is usual to use a mirror version of the version for adult users, i.e. the items that are present in the version for adult users, plus some items from the version for child users, are present in the version for health professionals (BRASIL, 2010b). In 2013, Hauser and colleagues completed the translation, adaptation and evaluation of the validity and reliability of the original version of the instrument for evaluating quality in PHC, for health professionals (HAUSER et al., 2013).

Even considering the regional differences and the large number of items (119), the PCATool-Brazil professional version captured the main attributes of PHC and generally showed acceptable reliability measures, given the reality in which the instrument was applied.

Thus, the PCATool-Brazil can be considered a valid and reliable instrument for assessing the presence and extent of PHC attributes in the experience of health professionals. It is therefore an important tool for evaluating health services, providing managers with information on the presence and extent of PHC attributes. For a detailed local assessment of the presence and extent of PHC attributes, we suggest using the PCATool-Brazil version for health professionals, whose validity and reliability were verified by Hauser and collaborators (2013). Although it is a somewhat extensive instrument, it allows us to specifically identify possible indicators of low quality that require action and/or monitoring (HAUSER et al., 2013).

Fracolli L. A. and collaborators (2014), in a *qualitative literature review followed by a meta-synthesis, identified instruments that have been used to evaluate Primary Health Care (PHC) and concluded that* the most suitable instrument is the PCATool, as it allows health care to be evaluated in its attributes, both essential and derived, in line with the PNAB proposal, which has Family Health as its priority strategy for expanding and consolidating PHC.

The PCATool prevails as the most widely used instrument in Brazil to evaluate PHC, due to its recognition, acceptance and validation in several countries such as the United States, Spain and others (FRACOLLI L. A. *et al.,* 2014).

At the national level, in 2010 the Ministry of Health published the Primary Health Care Evaluation Instrument Manual - PCATool-Brazil (BRASIL, 2010b), recognizing its importance and reliability in PHC evaluation processes. It also proposed criteria on elements of structure and process in order to guarantee quality in PHC services, through the Family Health Strategy Quality Improvement Assessment - AMQ and later the Program for Improving Access and Quality - PMAQ (HARZHEIM, et al. 2013).

The AMQ, a self-assessment instrument based on Donabedian's evaluation assumptions, was launched in 2008 with the aim of reinforcing the practice of continuous evaluation as an instrument for decision-making in the search for quality improvement. A study by Figueiredo (2011), which analyzed the agreement between the PCATool and AMQ instruments in the municipality of Curitiba, Paranà, suggests that, due to the lack of studies validating the AMQ and the low agreement between the two, the PCATool is the preferred tool for evaluating PHC.

The Ministry of Health currently uses the Self-Assessment for Improving Access and Quality in Primary Care (AMAQ) as part of its process of monitoring and evaluating processes and results, through the National Program for Improving Access and Quality in Primary Care (PMAQ) (BRASIL, 2012; BRASIL, 2013a).

The purpose of the PMAQ is to induce the expansion of access to and improvement of the quality of primary care, guaranteeing a standard of quality that is comparable nationally, regionally and locally, allowing for greater transparency and effectiveness of government actions directed at PHC (BRASIL, 2012; BRASIL, 2013a).

Among its specific objectives are the institutionalization of a culture of evaluation of PHC in the SUS and of management based on the induction and monitoring of processes and results, as well as stimulating the focus of PHC on the user, promoting the transparency of management processes, social participation and control and the health responsibility of health professionals and managers with the improvement of health conditions and user satisfaction. It is organized in four phases that complement each other, forming a continuous cycle of improving access to and quality of PHC, including self-evaluation, monitoring, continuing education and institutional support. There is also an external evaluation phase, which should offer certification to PHC teams and municipal managers, based on their performance, as well as evaluating user satisfaction (BRASIL, 2012; BRASIL, 2013a).

Evaluating the quality of PHC services in Brazil is essential, as the rapid expansion of these services, especially through the FHS, has been associated with several favorable outcomes, such as a reduction in infant mortality, a reduction in hospitalizations for PHC-sensitive conditions and advances in integration with the care network. Despite this, there are still weaknesses in access and integrality of care, making greater financial investment and expansion of services essential, identifying where the network still needs to be expanded and what adjustments need to be made to the existing structure (HARZHEIM, et al. 2013).

In recent decades, PHC has been evaluated in different ways in various countries. A comparison of 12 industrialized countries indicated that those with a stronger orientation towards PHC are more likely to have better levels of health and lower costs in this sector (STARFIELD, 2002).

A study by Shi (1994) in 50 states in the United States showed that the higher the number of primary care doctors and the lower the number of specialists, the lower the morbidity and mortality rates and the better the life expectancy of the population studied.

Other national studies show that a better result in terms of PHC attributes is related, among other factors, to better training and qualification of PHC professionals (CASTRO, 2012; CHOMATAS, 2013; KOLLING, 2008; VITÓRIA, 2013).

In a study by Kolling (2008), who evaluated factors associated with the quality of PHC services in 32 small municipalities in Rio Grande do Sul, in the perception of 198 doctors and nurses, he identified that the perception of capacity in specific PHC skills, such as multidisciplinary work, home visits, family and community approaches are strongly linked to a better quality of services, suggesting the importance of EPS in the qualification of professionals to work in PHC.

In a study to measure the presence and extent of PHC attributes in Curitiba in 2008, Chomatas et al. (2013) applied the PCATool to 490 doctors and nurses in 2008. The significant variables associated with a high PHC score were training in Family and Community Medicine or Community Nursing and the type of unit (ESF or traditional unit).

A study by Tesser and collaborators (2011), carried out in Florianópolis between 2007 and 2009 with professionals from the Family Health teams, through semi-structured interviews, points to the importance of continuing education for broadening the understanding and practice of health promotion in PHC.

Considering the importance of PHC and the significant expansion of the ESF, it is necessary to speed up the process of changes in the training and development of health workers. This is an issue directly related to the quality of PHC and requires the establishment of solid and lasting partnerships with training institutions. It is up to managers to identify demands that reflect the real needs of health services and that express the interests of society, breaking with practices where the market and corporate interests direct the process of training and specialization of health professionals (BRASIL, 2011b).

For these changes to take place, both in training and in PHC practices, the continuing education policy must contribute to improving the process of knowledge and analysis of social reality, as well as to increasing resolubility, longitudinality, humanization, coordination of care and pedagogical and cultural competence in health care (TESSER et al., 2011).

CHAPTER 6

METHODOLOGICAL PATH

This is a cross-sectional study carried out in the municipality of Goiânia, capital of the state of Goiás, from August to November 2013. The municipality has an estimated population of 1,412,364 inhabitants (IBGE, 2014), with the Health Care Network organized into seven regions, called Health Districts.

In 2012, the population of the municipality was approximately 1,302,001 inhabitants and in the northwest region 164,283 inhabitants (IBGE, 2012), which corresponds to 12.6% of the municipality's population at the time. Its Health Care Network is made up of 18 Family Health Centers (CSF), three Comprehensive Health Care Centers (CAIS), a Maternity Hospital, a technical and administrative unit (Distrito Sanitàrio), three NASFs and a Multiprofessional Home Care Team, all registered in the National Registry of Health Establishments (CNES). According to the 2016 PHC Planning calculations (BRASIL, 2011a), the region has 51% FHS coverage, with 51 Family Health teams made up of 53 doctors, 50 nurses, 21 dental surgeons, as well as oral health assistants, community health agents and nursing assistants.

A total of 53 doctors and 50 nurses working in the ESF in the northwestern region of Goiânia and working in the CSF during the data collection period were invited to take part in the study, totaling 103 professionals. Two professionals on medical leave during the data collection period were excluded from the study.

The sample was a convenience sample, totaling 101 professionals. There were two refusals and seven losses after five unsuccessful application attempts, resulting in a final sample of 92 participants.

The size of the sample studied made it possible to identify the association between having a specialization and a high PHC score, with a test power (β)

of 80% and a 95% confidence interval (CHOMATAS et al., 2013; HULLEY et al., 2001).

Data was collected through interviews. Two structured questionnaires were used:

> Questionnaire on the profile of academic training, professional qualifications and occupational characteristics, based on studies by Castro (2009; 2013), Chomatas (2009), Leâo and Caldeira (2011) and prepared by the researcher in charge.

> PCA-Tool Questionnaire - Primary Care Assessment Tool, version for professionals, validated in Brazil (BRASIL, 2010b; HAUSER et al., 2013).

The PCA Tool allows scores to be obtained for PHC attributes, in dimensions (first contact access, continued care/longitudinality, coordination and comprehensiveness), sub-dimensions (family approach/orientation, community orientation and cultural competence) and overall score (Chart 1).

The instrument's dimensions are structured according to a *Likert-type* scale, which assigns scores from 1 to 4 to the attribute (1 = definitely not, 2 = probably not, 3 = probably yes, 4 = definitely yes). The scores for each attribute are produced using the arithmetic mean of the items that make it up and converted into a scale from zero to ten. A score equal to or greater than 6.6, which comprises the upper tertile of the score, was considered a high PHC score (BRASIL, 2010b, HAUSER et al., 2013).

Chart 1: Primary Health Care Scores and Attributes

Score	Attributes	Description
Essential	First contact access or accessibility	Gateway to the health system, the first resource to be sought when there is a health need/problem

	Longitudinality or continuous care	A relationship of bonding and responsibility that is established over time between individuals and the health team, monitoring the various stages of the life cycle, as a regular source of care.
	Coordination of care Coordination Coordination (information systems)	Based on information and identification of the population's needs, multidisciplinary action and coordination of actions and responses to meet those needs.
	Comprehensive services available Services provided	Ability to deal with the wide range of health needs of the population, either by resolving them, or by arranging for them to receive any kind of care required.
Non-essential or	Family guidance or	It addresses the extent to which PHC focuses on the health of individuals in the context of the family, considering its
derived	focus on the family	potential for care and also as a threat to health, including the use of family approach tools
	Community orientation	It recognizes the health needs of the community through direct contact and epidemiological data, promoting joint planning and evaluation of services.
	Cultural competence	addresses relationships with people from different groups and cultures, seeking to value cultural characteristics, beliefs and values of the population in the

| | | relationship and communication between professionals and the community |
| General | All | It considers all attributes and reflects the quality of PHC services provided to the population. |

Data collection was organized based on a survey of the units' professional staff, managers, work shifts, telephone numbers, addresses, GPS location, definition of interview routes and schedules, transportation and means of communication.

The interviews were scheduled a priori by telephone, and when this wasn't enough, in person. One to five scheduling attempts were made with each professional.

To collect the data, an interviewer's manual was drawn up with general and specific guidelines for carrying out the interviews, as well as training for the interviewers, who were two students from the UFG Nutrition course and the researcher. A pilot study was then carried out with a professional from a Family Health Team in the south-western region of Goiânia to test the data collection process and instruments. This study contributed to adaptations in the form and language of the questionnaire about the interviewees' educational and professional profile, while keeping the PCATool in its original format.

For the statistical analysis, the independent variables of the study were gender, age, profession, length of time since graduation, completion and type of post-graduation, length of time working in the ESF and in the team; offer, participation and perception of training by the professionals (Chart 2). The outcome variable was the quality of PHC services, where a value of 6.6 or more is considered a high PHC score (BRASIL, 2010b).

Table 2: Independent variables in the study

Category	Variable	Description

Demographics	Sex	Male or Female
	Age	Median in years < 30 years or ≥ 30 years
Academic background	Profession	By professional category (doctor, nurse)
	Time since graduation	Median in years < 5 years or ≥ 5 years
	Type of Educational Institution	Public or Private
Postgraduate	Postgraduate degree	Yes or No
	Type of Postgraduate Degree	*Latu* and *strictu senso* postgraduate levels (specialization, residency, master's and doctorate)
	Postgraduate Area	Related to PHC: Yes or No, where Yes: family health, public health, collective health, family and community medicine, general practice, pediatrics, gynecology-obstetrics.
Experience Professional	Time at experience in the ESF	Median in years < 2 years or ≥ 2 years
	Length of service in the team	Median in years < 1 year or ≥ 1 year
Participation in Training	Participation in training	Yes or No (in the last 12 months, related to ESF activities)
	Type of training carried out	Training modalities: Short and medium-term courses (up to 60 hours), In-service training Events (Congresses, Seminars, Forums, Exhibitions, etc.)

Contribution of training to	Professional development Changes in professional practice	Conversion of *Likert* scale into Yes or No category, where: Yes: a little, a lot, extremely No: nothing, neutral

The data was double-entered into the EPI INFO software (version 6.04), and the databases were checked for consistency using *Validate*. The data was processed using the statistical program Stata version SE.64. A 5% significance level was adopted for statistical analysis.

The *Swilk* test was used to check the distribution of the data. After identifying the variables that did not show normal distribution, the *Man-Whitney U-test* for continuous variables and Pearson's chi-square or Fischer's test for categorical variables were used to analyze the independent variables and the PCATool attributes and scores.

In order to identify the variables which, at the level of the professional, are associated with a high overall PHC score, Pearson's chi-square or Fischer's tests were first used. The multivariate model included the independent variables that were individually shown to be associated with a high overall PHC score with a p-value < 0.30. Poisson regression with robust variance was performed, and the prevalence ratio (PR) with its confidence intervals (CI) was presented as the measure of effect. Subsequently, the variables with the highest p-values were excluded, so that only those with p-values < 0.05 remained in the final model.

In all its stages, this research took into account the fundamental ethical principles that guide research involving human beings, described and established by the National Health Council Resolution No. 466 of December 12, 2012 (BRASIL, 2013b).

The project was approved by the Research Ethics Committee of the Hospital das Clinicas da UFG, under substantiated opinion No. 336.524/2013.

CHAPTER 7

TRAINING AND QUALIFICATION OF PROFESSIONALS: FACTORS ASSOCIATED WITH THE QUALITY OF PRIMARY HEALTH CARE SERVICES

Of the 101 eligible professionals, 92 (91.1%) took part in the study, 48 (52.2%) of whom were doctors and 44 (47.8%) nurses. The training profile, professional experience and qualifications of the professionals interviewed can be seen in Table 1.

Table 1. Demographic characteristics, education profile, professional experience and qualifications of doctors and nurses at Family Health Strategy units in the northwest region of Goiânia, 2013.

Variables[T]	Total	Doctors	Nurses	p-value[f]
	92 (100%) n (%)	48 (52,2%) n (%)	44 (47,8%) n (%)	
Sex				
Male	25 (27,2)	22 (45,8)	3 (6,8)	<0,001
Female	67 (72,8)	26 (54,2)	41 (93,2)	
Age (years) [T]	35,4 (28,4-41,7)	28,9 (26,4-36,7)	38,2 (32,9-43,9)	<0,001
Age (age group)				
< 30 years	34 (37,0)	26 (54,2)	8 (18,2)	<0,001
≥ 30 years	58 (63,0)	22 (45,8)	36 (81,8)	
Academic Background **Time since graduation (years)** [T]	6,1 (1,9-13,7)	2,3 (0,9-5,9)	12,3 (6,8-15,6)	<0,001
Time since graduation				
< 5 years	41 (44,6)	35 (72,9)	6 (13,6)	<0,001
≥ 5 years	51 (55,4)	13 (27,1)	38 (86,4)	
Type of educational institution				
Public	40 (43,5)	21 (43,8)	19 (43,2)	0,956
Private	52 (56,5)	27 (56,2)	25 (56,8)	
Postgraduate				
Has a specialization				
Yes	55 (59,8)	17 (35,4)	38 (86,4)	<0,001
No	37 (40,2)	31 (64,6)	6 (13,6)	
Specialization Related to PHC [tt]				
Yes	37 (67,3)	10 (58,8)	27 (71,0)	0,372
No	18 (32,7)	7 (41,2)	11 (29,0)	

***Professional Experience* Time in the ESF (years)** [T]	3,4 (0,8-8,5)	1,35 (0,6-3,9)	7,3 (2,4-10,3)	<0,001
Time in the ESF < 2 years	39 (42,4)	29 (60,4)	10 (22,74)	<0,001
≥ 2 years	53 (57,6)	19 (39,6)	34 (77,3)	
Time in the Team (years) [T]	1,5 (0,5-4,5)	0,6 (0,3-1,5)	3,6 (1,3-5,5)	<0,001
Time in the Team				
< 1 year	38 (41,3)	30 (62,5)	8 (18,2)	<0,001
≥ 1 year		54 (58,7)	18 (37,5)	36 (81,8)
Participation in Training				
Participated in training				
Yes	78 (84,8)	40 (83,3)	38 (86,4)	0,686
No	14 (15,2)	8 (16,7)	6 (13,6)	
Participation Courses (up to 60 h) [ttt]	72 (92,3)	38 (95,0)	34 (89,5)	0,425
Participation in in-service training [ttt]	54 (69,3)	26 (65,0)	28 (73,7)	0,406
Participation in Events [ttt]	46 (59,0)	23 (60,5)	23 (57,5)	0,786
Contribution of Capacities for: [ttt]				
Professional development	75 (96,2)	38 (95,0)	37 (97,4)	1,000
Changes in professional practice	69 (88,5)	34 (85,0)	35 (92,1)	0,482

[T] Continuous variables are presented as median and interquartile range (p25- p75).

[i] Obtained using the Man-Whitney U-test for continuous variables and the chi-square or Fischer tests for categorical variables.

[tt] Only individuals who reported having completed a postgraduate course were considered (doctors n=17; nurses n=38, total n=55).

[ttt] Only individuals who reported having undergone training were considered (doctors n=40; nurses n=38, total n=78). Different types of training may have been carried out in the period by the same professional.

The study group was made up of 67 (72.8%) women, with a predominance of this profile in both professional categories, especially among nurses (n=41; 93.2%).

The median age (interquartile range 25-75) of the professionals was 35.4 (28.4-41.7) years, with 28.9 (26.4-36.7) years for doctors and 38.2 (32.9-43.9) years for nurses (p<0.001). In terms of age groups, 58 (63.0%) professionals were aged 30 or over, with a greater distribution among nurses (n=36; 81.8%) than among doctors (n=22; 45.8%) (p<0.001).

The median length of academic training was 6.1 (1.9-13.7) years. Among doctors it was 2.3 (0.9-5.9) years, while for nurses it was 12.3 (6.8-15.6) years, with a statistically significant difference (p<0.001). The proportion of nurses with more than five years of training (n=38; 86.4%) was also significantly higher than that of doctors (n=13; 27.1%), (p<0.001).

As for the institution where they were trained, 21 (43.8%) doctors and 19 (43.2%) nurses reported that they were trained in a public institution (p>0.05).

Specialization was reported by 55 (59.8%) professionals, 17 (35.4%) of whom were doctors and 38 (86.4%) nurses, indicating a significant predominance of postgraduate studies among nurses (p<0.001). Of the professionals who had completed postgraduate studies, 37 (67.3%) reported having a specialty in PHC, with no significant difference between the professional categories.

The time spent working in the FHS and in the same team showed overall medians 3.4 (0.8-8.5) and 1.5 (0.5-4.5) years. Both were significantly longer for nurses than for doctors (p<0.001). More than half of the doctors have been working in the FHS for less than a year, unlike the nurses (p<0.001).

78 (84.8%) professionals reported having undergone training related to their activities in the FHS in the last year, with a similar percentage between doctors and nurses. Of these, 72 (92.3%) reported courses of up to 60 hours as the main training strategy, followed by in-service training (n=54; 69.3%) and participation in events such as congresses, seminars, symposiums, etc. (n=46; 59%), with no statistically significant differences between the professional categories.

The majority of professionals who took part in training said that it contributed both to professional development (n=75; 96.2%) and to changes in professional practice and/or quality of service (n=69; 88.5%).

The presence and extent of PHC attributes considering the average scores and the presence of a high PHC score (≥6.6) for each attribute, essential score, non-essential score and overall PHC score are shown in Table 2.

Table 2. Mean (SD) scores [t] of the attributes and essential, non-essential and general scores of primary health care and frequency (%) of high scores (≥ 6.6) in the evaluation of doctors and nurses from the Family Health Strategy units in the northwest region of Goiânia, 2013.

Attributes	Average scores (SD) n=92	High score (≥6.6)			
		Total n (%) 92 (100)	Doctor n (%) 48 (52.2)	Nurse n (%) 44 (47.8)	p-value[ii]
First contact - access	4,6±1,0	5 (5,4)	3 (6,3)	2 (4,5)	1,000
Longitudinality	6,8±1,2	53 (57,6)	29 (60,4)	24 (54,5)	0,569
Coordination	6,9±1,3	57 (62,0)	36 (75,0)	21 (47,7)	0,007
Coordination (information systems)	6,5±1,4	50 (54,4)	29 (60,4)	21 (47,7)	0,222
Comprehensiveness (services available)	6,5±1,4	49 (53,3)	26 (54,2)	23 (52,3)	0,856
Comprehensiveness (services provided)	8,0±1,4	78 (84,8)	39 (81,3)	39 (88,6)	0,324
Essential Score	6,5±0,9	44 (47,8)	26 (54,2)	18 (40,9)	0,204
Focus on the family	7,6±1,6	67 (72,8)	36 (75,0)	31 (70,5)	0,624
Community orientation	6,5±1,4	45 (48,9)	24 (50,0)	21 (47,7)	0,828
Cultural competence	6,6±2,0	44 (47,8)	22 (45,8)	22 (50,0)	0,689
Derived Score (Non-Essential)	6,9±1,4	77 (83,7)	41 (85,4)	36 (81,8)	0,641
Overall score	6,7±1,0	52 (56,5)	29 (60,4)	23 (52,3)	0,431

[t]Scores take values from 0 to 10, where values ≥ 6.6 indicate a high PHC score. [tt]Obtained by chi-square or Fischer's test.

The overall average PHC score obtained by PCATool-Brazil was 6.7 (±1.0), which is considered a high PHC score, but close to the cut-off point (≥6.6). 52 (56.5%) professionals contributed to the high PHC score, of which 29 (60.4%) were doctors and 23 (52.3) were nurses.

The average essential PHC score was 6.5 (±0.9), identified as a low PHC score. The score for first contact access was the lowest, at 4.6 (±1.0), and the highest was Comprehensiveness/services provided (8.0±1.4). The proportion of high essential PHC scores was 47.8% (n= 44), of which 26 (54.2%) were doctors and 18 (40.9%) nurses.

The analysis of the non-essential attributes resulted in a high score of 6.9 (±1.4), where only the community orientation attribute had a low PHC score (6.5±1.4). The opinion of 77 (83.7%) professionals, of whom 41 (85.4%) were doctors and 36 (81.8%) nurses, resulted in a high non-essential PHC score.

After analyzing the mean scores between doctors and nurses, no significant differences were identified between the professional categories.

The profile of high PHC scores was also similar between the categories, with the exception of coordination of care, which showed a statistically significant difference, indicating a higher proportion of high PHC scores for doctors in this attribute.

Table 3 shows that there was no significant association between the presence of a high PHC score and the training and qualification profile of the professionals. However, in an analysis by professional category (data not shown), it was identified that, for doctors, working in the same team for a period of one year or more and the perception that training contributed to professional improvement were associated with a high PHC score ($p<0.05$).

Table 3. Association between the presence of a high general PHC score and its predictors among doctors and nurses working in the Family Health Strategy in the north-western region of Goiânia, Goiás.

Predictors	Low score n=40 (43.5%)	High score n=52 (56.5%)	p-value [τ]
Sex			
Male	11 (27,5)	14 (26,9)	0,951
Female	29 (72,5)	38 (73,1)	
Age	15 (37,5)	19 (36,5)	
< 30 years			0,925
≥ 30 years			
Academic background			
Profession	25 (62,5)	33 (63,5)	
Doctor	19 (39,6)	29 (60,4)	0,431
Nurse	21 (47,7)	23 (52,3)	
Time since graduation	15 (37,5)	22 (42,3)	
< 5 years			0,641
≥ 5 years			
Type of training institution	25 (62,5)	30 (57,7)	
Public	19 (47,5)	21 (40,4)	0,495
Private	21 (52,5)	31 (59,6)	
Has a specialization	13 (32,5)	24 (46,2)	
No			0,185
Yes	27 (67,5)	28 (53,8)	
Specialization Related to PHC[n]	9 (33,3)	9 (32,1)	
No			0,925
Yes	18 (66,7)	19 (67,9)	
***Professional Experience* Time working in the ESF**	15 (37,5)	24 (46,2)	
< 2 years			0,405
≥ 2 years	25 (62,5)	28 (51,8)	
Time working in the team	18 (45,0)	20 (38,5)	
< 1 year			0,528
≥ 1 year			
Training			
Participated in training	22 (55,0)	32 (61,5)	
No	8 (20,0)	6 (11,5)	0,263
Yes	32 (80,0)	46 (88,5)	
Courses (up to 60 h)[^ τ^ τ^(τ)]	3 (9,4)	3 (6,5)	
No			0,645
Yes	29 (90,6)	43 (93,5)	
In-service training [τττ] No	11 (34,4)	13 (28,3)	0,565
Yes	21 (65,6)	33 (71,7)	
Events [τττ]			
No	14 (43,8)	18 (39,1)	0,683

Yes	18 (56,2)	28 (60,9)	
Contribution of training to: [TTT]			
Professional development	29 (90,6)	46 (100,0)	0,065
Changes in practice	27 (84,4)	42 (91,3)	0,475

[T] Chi-square or Fischer's test.

[TT] Only individuals who reported having completed a postgraduate course were considered (doctors n=17; nurses n=38, total n=55).

[TTT] Only individuals who reported having undergone training were considered (doctors n=40; nurses n=38, total n=78). Different types of training may have been carried out in the period by the same professional.

Table 4 shows the regression analysis used to define a final explanatory model, showing no association between the selected variables and the high PHC score in the general model.

Table 4: Adjusted Model [t] of the High General Value of PHC among doctors and nurses from the Family Health Strategy in the northwestern region of Goiânia, 2013.

Variables	PR (95% CI)	p-value
Specialization No	1	0,143
Yes	0,59 (0,29-1,20)	
Training held No	1	0,153
Yes	1,76 (0,81-3,81)	
Professional Development No	1	0,151
Yes	0,78 (0,56-1,09)	

[+] Poisson regression.

CHAPTER 8

DO TRAINING AND QUALIFICATIONS INFLUENCE THE QUALITY OF PRIMARY HEALTH CARE?

The results of this study show that, in the northwestern region of Goiânia, the quality of PHC services in the ESF is satisfactory in the perception of doctors and nurses, and that nurses have more experience, professional qualifications and ties to the ESF than doctors, training contributes to improvement and changes in professional practice and that the profile of training and qualification of professionals is associated with the longer time doctors have worked in the same team and with the perception of training of health professionals in the northwest region of Goiânia.

The proportion of losses in the sample (8.9%) was within expectations, considering similar studies that describe the profile of professionals and analyze the quality of services through the PCATool, version for professionals: 7.9% (CASTRO et al., 2012; HAUSER et al., 2013), 15% (VITÓRIA et al., 2013) and 28% (CHOMATAS et al., 2013).

The identification of the professionals' profile showed that the doctors are younger, have been trained for less time, have a lower proportion of postgraduate degrees and have worked for the ESF and the team for less time; a profile similar to that found in other states and regions of Brazil (MACHADO et al., 2000; TOMASI et al., 2008).

The predominance of women in the health sector is confirmed in most studies, especially among nurses (HAUSER et al., 2013; KOLLING, 2008; MACHADO, 2000; ROCHA, 2008; TOMASI et al., 2008). Studies on the profile of health professionals in Brazil conclude that today's medicine is experiencing changes in professional practice. These include rejuvenation and the rapid and irreversible feminization of the medical field (FERRARI; THOMSON; MELCHIOR, 2005). This study found that doctors under the age of 30 who are female represent more than half of the entire medical profession.

With regard to PHC attributes, the overall score in this study was satisfactory, but close to the cut-off point for a high PHC score and lower than the majority of similar studies carried out in southern Brazil (CASTRO et al., 2012; CHOMATAS et al., 2013; KOLLING, 2008; VITÓRIA et al., 2013). An important aspect is that almost half of the professionals reported a low overall PHC score, demonstrating that there is still a lot to improve in the quality of these services, in order to guarantee not only the presence, but a wide range of attributes.

In most similar studies, first contact access is the attribute with the lowest average score (CASTRO et al., 2012; CHOMATAS et al., 2013; KOLLING, 2008; VITÓRIA et al., 2013). In the present study, in addition to the low score for the access attribute contributing to the reduction in the overall score, only 5% of the professionals reported that the service had satisfactory accessibility, which may be related to the low availability of services to citizens in relation to the needs of the area, which has a high pent-up demand for care and an overload of emergency services.

In a study with users and health professionals carried out in Petrópolis (RJ), the results obtained by health professionals were higher in terms of access when compared to users, suggesting that in the perception of professionals, access is better than in the opinion of users, who experience the barriers of first contact with the health system on a daily basis (MACINKO; ALMEIDA; SA, 2007).

The Integrality attribute, related to the services provided, obtained a high PHC score in the perception of the majority of interviewees, coinciding with the majority of studies (CASTRO et al., 2012; CHOMATAS et al., 2013; KOLLING, 2008; VITÓRIA et al., 2013) and indicating that professionals feel prepared and sensitive to addressing the most diverse health problems, considering their risk factors and social determinants. However, this result contrasts with the results of another aspect of comprehensiveness, the services available, whose score was low. Looking at the PCATool questions, the results show that professionals have a good self-assessment of their approach from the perspective of comprehensiveness, but suggest that management does not offer adequate working conditions and a portfolio of services to guarantee comprehensiveness through the services available.

The attribute Coordination of care showed better results among doctors, who may have interpreted the questions as knowledge, actions and coordination of the flow of specialized consultations, such as referral and counter-referral, which although it is the responsibility of doctors and nurses, in the municipality of Goiânia it is mainly carried out by doctors. However, it is known that nurses play a fundamental role in coordinating the Family Health Centers, both in administrative, technical, pedagogical and care aspects (ROCHA, 2008).

The lack of association between the training and qualification profile of professionals and the quality of ESF services, in the general model, suggests that the challenges of consolidating PHC have their roots in the process of training professionals, which, despite efforts to change and advances in the concepts and programs of higher education in health in Brazil, is still far removed from the needs of the SUS, especially the ESF. Most medical schools still focus their teaching on hospitals and diseases, making the training apparatus disconnected from the communities and health services associated with them (GOMES et al., 2012).

In traditional health training, curricula are more closed, tend to be less interdisciplinary and more specialized, leading to a fragmented study of people's and societies' health problems and hindering efficient teamwork. The training is little recognized by professionals as belonging to primary care, seen "as medicine for the poor", far from the hospital's accolade and scientific aura. As for the pedagogical approach, it is often limited to traditional methodologies based on the transmission of knowledge, which do not favor the critical formation of the student (ALMEIDA FILHO, 2013; BRASIL, 2007a; 2011b;

GOMES et al., 2012).

According to Gomes et al. (2012), the main problems associated with the training of professionals are the dissociation between theory and practice, the mismatch between the basic-clinical cycles, the antagonism between clinical and collective health, specialists *versus* generalists, the lack of training to deal with the majority of people's problems, dehumanization, among others.

To overcome these shortcomings, professional training in PHC can be stimulated through programs to strengthen and reorient the process of training and developing human resources in the health area, such as the National Program for Reorienting Professional Training in Health (PRO-Saùde) (BRASIL, 2007a) and the Education through Work for Health Program (PET-Saùde) (BRASIL, 2010c), projects that aim to integrate teaching, service and community, through the inclusion of teachers and undergraduate students in the public health network, with a view to professional training with a comprehensive approach to the health-disease process with an emphasis on primary care.

These initiatives towards curriculum integration and the proposal to diversify teaching-learning scenarios in undergraduate medical schools have been gaining prominence in health education. In fact, the opportunity to work in different settings is now a fundamental aspect of training doctors to work more closely with individuals and society, as well as making learning meaningful (GOMES et al., 2012).

With regard to postgraduate studies, it can be seen that, in general, specialization in different areas related to PHC is consistent with what has been observed in the literature (CASTRO et al., 2012; CHOMATAS et al., 2013; HAUSER et al., 2013; KOLLING, 2008; ROCHA, 2008; VITÓRIA et al., 2013). The significant difference in specialization between doctors and nurses may be related to the younger age and time since graduation of doctors, who, for the most part, are recent university graduates and have not yet started or completed postgraduate studies.

There is a tendency towards specialization in the health area, which has been pointed out, among other factors, as one of the factors responsible for the rise in healthcare costs and the poor geographical distribution of professionals in this area, to the detriment of PHC. This is not to deny the importance of specialization, but it is essential to seek a balance in the ratio of specialists to generalists, without jeopardizing the quality of care provided (BRASIL, 2007a).

Maciel et al. (2010), when evaluating the contribution of specialization in Family Health to the reorientation of health practices in the ESF, in Espirito Santo, in the perception of students who graduated from this course, were able to highlight the importance of post-graduation for professional qualification and changes in practice in the ESF, with reflexes in the improvement of services provided to the population.

In Goiânia, some Higher Education Institutions (HEIs), in partnership with the SMS, through the Ministries of Health and Education, have offered the municipality's health professionals free courses, some even paid, in the area of PHC, such as Specializations and Multiprofessional Residencies in Family Health (UFG) and the Family and Community Medicine Residency (Pontifical Catholic University of Goiàs - PUC Goiàs) (ROCHA, 2008).

Although he recognizes the importance of specializations, Minayo (2010) states that it is very difficult to distinguish the specific contribution of postgraduate studies to the consolidation of the SUS, because it involves several actors, such as teachers, researchers and their students, both personally and institutionally, as well as those who formulate policies and those who are responsible for their management.

In relation to professional experience, the effects of the training and qualification of professionals may explain, in part, the high turnover of doctors in the ESF and the better evaluation of the quality of PHC for doctors who stay longer in the ESF. The literature shows that it is difficult to introduce new professionals to the PHC proposal, as the majority who work in the system are still trained in a privatized, hospital-centric and overspecialized care model, leading to the political and social devaluation of PHC, which faces many challenges in becoming hegemonic as a proposal capable of confronting the existing fragmented model (BRASIL, 2011b).

On the other hand, the dynamism of opportunities in the job market for doctors in the most economically active regions can contribute to the voluntary resignation of doctors, who easily relocate in the job market (NEGRI, 2002).

A study carried out in Canada by Geneau et al. (2007) shows that the possible causes of the high turnover of doctors who work as gatekeepers to the health system are related to job dissatisfaction, such as increased workload, daily pressures and the withdrawal of professional autonomy.

In Curitiba, Paranà, the profile of FHS doctors seems to differ from what was observed in this study and in the national literature in general. ESF doctors are apparently more experienced than nurses, with an average age of 46.6 years, low turnover and a long time since graduation (17.8 years) (CHOMATAS et al., 2013), while in this study it was 2.3 years.

The provision of training was shown to be a positive aspect of the ESF in the northwestern region of Goiânia, as the majority of professionals reported having participated in training related to their activities in the last year, similar to the study in Curitiba (CHOMATAS et al., 2013), which has been used as a reference for the PHC model in this work (PAHO, 2013).

The results also indicate that the training courses have contributed significantly to the professional development of the interviewees, and that this has reflected in their professional practice or in a better quality of service, in the perception of the professionals.

In the study by Kolling (2008), which measured the experience of doctors and nurses with the FHS in 32 municipalities in Rio Grande do Sul, positive self-assessment of specific PHC skills (multidisciplinary work, home visits, family and community approaches) was significantly associated with a high overall PHC score, indicating that improving these skills, guided by the attributes of PHC, can be useful in achieving greater orientation among professionals in this proposal.

However, further studies are needed to clarify the principles and teaching-learning strategies that guide these training courses, with a view to contributing to the implementation of the PNEPS. According to Tesser (2011), EPS is a privileged instrument for analyzing reality, building health promotion actions, care in the ESF and overcoming the hierarchical and authoritarian view of education and work processes, thus qualifying the training and practices of PHC health professionals.

The association between the length of time working in the team and the perception of training with the quality of PHC demonstrates the importance of linking strategies and the qualification of professionals, from the perspective of EPS, in order to obtain better results in the evaluation of their attributes and, consequently, positive repercussions on the quality of the services provided to the population (CASTRO et al., 2012; KOLLING, 2008).

It is suggested that other factors may have influenced the results presented, such as changes in the political and economic scenario in the municipality, which reflect on public policies in the field of working conditions, safety, human, physical and material resources in the northwest region and the different conceptions and level of acceptance of health evaluation models.

The study's limitations include the use of a training and qualification profile instrument, which did not allow us to identify the pedagogical proposals and characteristics of the professionals' training and qualification, which could shed light on some aspects of their contribution to the quality of the services. As for the PCATool, it does not consider the structural evaluation of the service, as suggested by Vitória et al. (2013) and uses equal weights for the attributes in the measure of PHC orientation. The version of the instrument chosen for this study only considered measuring the degree of orientation towards PHC by evaluating the experience of professionals, and no measurement was made of the perception of users in relation to the attributes.

We can also recognize the limitations of this type of research, which is evaluative and cross-sectional and could be minimized through complementary studies with a qualitative focus.

It should be emphasized that this study is the first in the municipality of Goiânia to relate the training and qualification profile of health professionals to the quality of PHC services, using an evaluation method validated nationally and internationally and endorsed by the Ministry of Health and world literature.

CHAPTER 9

CONCLUSION

In the north-western region of Goiânia, in relation to the profile of the professionals, the majority are women, the doctors are younger, have been trained for less time, have a lower proportion of post-graduate degrees and have worked for the ESF for less time. On the other hand, the nurses in the team have more experience and professional qualifications, and are more closely linked to the ESF. The majority take part in training courses in their area of work and these have contributed to improvement and changes in professional practice.

The evaluation of the quality of PHC services shows a satisfactory process in relation to the non-essential score, but weak in the essential score, resulting in a high overall PHC score, but with indications that there is much to improve in the quality of these services.

The study concluded that there was an association between the qualification profile of professionals and the quality of PHC services in the stratified model, where, for doctors, working in the same team for a period of one year or more and the perception that training contributes to professional development were associated with a high PHC score. However, there was no association in the general model (doctors and nurses).

It should be emphasized that the evidence presented in this study has contributed to the management of human resources, with a view to guaranteeing the best quality of these services. However, further studies are needed to clarify the principles and teaching-learning strategies that guide the training provided, with a view to contributing to the implementation of the PNEPS, on the understanding that investment in training, with an emphasis on the principles of permanent education, can help to improve the quality of the services provided.

be a strategy for qualifying PHC. On the other hand, it is suggested that new evaluations be carried out which take into account the perception of users, for example by means of the PCATool-Brazil version for users.

REFERENCES

ALMEIDA FILHO, N. M. de. Contexts, impasses and challenges in the training of workers in Collective Health in Brazil. **Ciência & saùde coletiva**, Rio de Janeiro, v. 18, n. 6, p. 1677-1682, jun. 2013. Disponivel em: <http://dx.doi.org/10.1590/S1413-81232013000600019>. Accessed on: July 3, 2017.

ALMEIDA, C.; MACINKO, J. **Validation of a methodology for rapid evaluation of the organizational characteristics and performance of primary care services of the health system (SUS) at the local level**. Brasilia: Pan American Health Organization. Technical series on the development of health systems and services, v.10, 2006. 215p.

AQUINO, R.; OLIVEIRA, N.; BARRETO, M. Impact of the family health program on infant mortality in Brazilian municipalities. **American Journal of Public Health**, v. 99, n. 1, p. 87-93, jan. 2009. Available at: <https://www.ncbi.nlm.nih.gov/pmc/articles/PMC2636620/>. Accessed on: July 3, 2017.

BRAZIL. National Council of Health Secretaries. **Primary Care and Health Promotion**. Brasilia: CONASS, 2011b. 197 p.

BRAZIL. National Council of Health Secretaries. **Planning Primary Health Care in the States**. Brasilia : CONASS, 2011a. 436 p.

BRAZIL. **Constitution (1988)**. Brasilia, DF: Senado Federal: Centro Gràfico, 1988. 292 p.

BRAZIL. Law No. 8080 of September 19, 1990. Provides for the conditions for the promotion, protection and recovery of health, the organization and financing of the corresponding services and other measures. **Official Gazette of the Federative Republic of Brazil**, Brasilia, DF, September 29, 1990.

BRAZIL. Law No. 9394 of December 20, 1996. Provides for the Guidelines and Bases of National Education. **Official Gazette of the Federative Republic of**

Brazil, Brasilia, DF, Dec. 23, 1996.

BRAZIL. Ministry of Education. Ministerial Opinion No. 1133 of August 7, 2001. Deliberates on the National Curriculum Guidelines for Degree Courses in Nursing, Medicine and Nutrition. **Official Gazette of the Federative Republic of Brazil**, Brasilia, DF, October 3, 2001.

BRAZIL. Ministry of Health. National Health Council. **Principios e Diretrizes para NOB/RH-SUS**. 2. ed. Brasilia: Ministério da Saùde, 2003.

BRAZIL. Ministry of Health. National Health Council. Resolution No. 466 of December 12, 2012. Guidelines and regulatory standards for research involving human beings. **Diàrio Oficial da Repùblica Federativa do** Brasil, Brasilia, DF, n. 12, 13 jun. 2013b.

BRAZIL. Ministry of Health. Ministry of Education. *Interministerial Ordinance No. 610 of March 26, 2002. Institutes the National Program to Encourage Curricular Changes in Medical Schools - Promed.*

Official Gazette of the Federative Republic of Brazil, Brasilia, DF, April 27, 2002.

BRAZIL. Ministry of Health. Ministry of Education. *Interministerial Ordinance No. 2.101 of November 3, 2005.* Institutes the National Program for the Reorientation of Professional Training in Health - Pró-Saùde - for undergraduate courses in Medicine, Nursing and Dentistry.

Official Gazette of the Federative Republic of Brazil, Brasilia, DF, 2005.

BRAZIL. Ministry of Health. Ministry of Education. *Interministerial Ordinance No. 421 of March 3, 2010.* Establishes the Work Education Program for Health (PET Health) and makes other provisions. **Official Gazette of the Federative Republic of Brazil,** Brasilia, DF, March 5, 2010c.

BRAZIL. Ministry of Health. Ministry of Education. **National Program for the Reorientation of Professional Training in Health. Pró-Saùde: objectives, implementation and potential development**. Brasilia: Ministry of Health,

2007a. 86 p.

BRAZIL. Ministry of Health. Ministerial Ordinance 198 of February 2004. Institutes the National Policy for Permanent Education in Health as a strategy of the Unified Health System for the training and development of workers for the sector and makes other provisions. **Diàrio Oficial da Repùblica Federativa do** Brasil, Brasilia, DF, n. 32/ 2004, secçâo I, 2004a.

BRAZIL. Ministry of Health. Ordinance No. 1.996, of August 20, 2007. Provides guidelines for the implementation of the National Policy for Permanent Education in Health and other measures. **Official Gazette of the Federative Republic of Brazil**, Brasilia, DF, Aug. 22, 2007b.

BRAZIL. Ministry of Health. Ordinance No. 2.048, of September 3, 2009. Approves the Regulations of the Unified Health System (SUS). **Official Gazette of the Federative Republic of Brazil**, Brasilia, DF, September 4, 2009b.

BRAZIL. Ministry of Health. Ordinance No. 2.488, of October 21, 2011. Approves the National Primary Care Policy and makes other provisions.

Official Gazette of the Federative Republic of Brazil, Brasilia, DF, October 24, 2011c.

BRAZIL. Ministry of Health. Health Care Secretariat. Department of Primary Care. **National Primary Care Policy**. Health Pact Series 2006. Brasilia: Ministry of Health, 2006. 60 p.

BRAZIL. Ministry of Health. Health Care Secretariat. Department of Primary Care. **NASF Guidelines**. Cadernos de Atençâo Bàsica, n. 27. Brasilia: Ministério da Saùde, 2010a. 160 p.

BRAZIL. Ministry of Health. Health Care Secretariat. Department of Primary Care. **National Program for Improving Access and Quality in Primary Care (PMAQ): instructional manual / Ministry of Health**. Brasilia: Ministry of Health, 2012. 62 p.

BRAZIL. Ministry of Health. Health Care Secretariat. Department of Primary Care. **Self-assessment to improve access to and quality of primary care - Family Health Support Centers - AMAQ - NASF**. Brasilia: Ministry of Health, 2013a. 66 p.

BRAZIL. Ministry of Health. Health Care Secretariat.

Department of Primary Care. **Manual for the primary health care assessment tool pcatool - Brazil**. Brasilia: Ministry of Health, 2010b. 80p.

BRAZIL. Ministry of Health. Secretariat for Labor Management and Health Education. Department of Health Education Management.

AprenderSUS: the SUS and undergraduate health courses. Brasilia: Ministry of Health, 2004b. 20 p.

BRAZIL. Ministry of Health. Secretariat for Labor Management and Health Education. Department of Health Education Management.

Politica de educaçao e desenvolvimento para o SUS: caminhos para a educaçao permanente em saù: pólos de educaçao permanente em saù. Brasilia: Ministry of Health, 2004c. 68 p.

BRAZIL. Ministry of Health. Secretariat for Labor Management and Health Education. Department of Health Education Management.

National Policy for Permanent Education in Health. Series Pactos pela Saùde 2006. Brasilia: Ministry of Health, 2009a. v. 9. 64 p.

CARDOSO, I. M.; MURAD, A. G.; BOF, S. M. S. The institutionalization of permanent education in the family health program: an innovative municipal experience. **Trabalho, educaçâo e saùde** [online], v. 3, n. 2, p. 429440, 2005. Available at:< http://dx.doi.org/10.1590/S1981- 77462005000200010>. Accessed on: July 3, 2017.

CASTRO, R. C. L. et al. Evaluation of the quality of primary care by health professionals: comparison between different types of services.

Cadernos de Saùblica, Rio de Janeiro, v. 28, n. 9, 2012. Available at: <http://dx.doi.org/10.1590/S0102-311X2012000900015> . Accessed on: 03 jul. 2017.

CASTRO, R. C. L. **Percepção dos profissionais médicos e enfermeiros sobre a qualidade da Atenção à Saúde do adulto: comparação entre os serviços de Atenção Primària de Porto Alegre**. Porto Alegre: FAMED/ HCPA Library, 2009. Available at: http://hdl.handle.net/10183/18766. Accessed on: June 23, 2017.

CECCIM, R. B. Permanent Education in Health: decentralization and dissemination of pedagogical capacity in health. **Ciência & Saùde Coletiva**, Rio de Janeiro, v. 10, n. 4, dec. 2005. Available at: <http://dx.doi.org/10.1590/S1413-81232005000400020> . Accessed on: July 3, 2017.

CECCIM, R. B.; FERLA, A. A. Educaçâo e saùde: ensino e cidadania como travessia de fronteiras. **Trabalho, educaçâo e saùde**, Rio de Janeiro, v. 6, n. 3, 2008. Available at:< http://dx.doi.org/10.1590/S1981-77462008000300003>. Accessed on: July 3, 2017.

CECCIM, R. B.; FEUERWERKER, L. C. M. The quadrilateral of training for the health area: teaching, management, care and social control. **Physis - Revista Saùde Coletiva**, v. 14, n. 1, p. 41-65, 2004. Available at: <http://hdl.handle.net/10183/27642>. Accessed on: July 3, 2017.

CHOMATAS, E. et al. Evaluation of the presence and extent of primary care attributes in Curitiba. **Revista Brasileira de Medicina de Familia e Comunidade**, Rio de Janeiro, v. 8, n. 29, p. 294-303, Oct/Dec. 2013.

Available at: <http://hdl.handle.net/10183/139094>. Accessed on: July 3, 2017.

CHOMATAS, E. R. V. **Avaliação da presença e extensão dos atributos da Atenção Primària na rede bàsica de saúde no município de Curitiba, no ano de 2008**. Porto Alegre: Biblioteca FAMED/ HCPA, 2009. Available at:

http://www.lume.ufrgs.br/bitstream/handle/10183/24606/000747716.pdf?sequ
ence=1. Accessed on: June 24, 2014.

NATIONAL HEALTH CONFERENCE, 8ª, 1987, Brasilia. **Proceedings of the
8th National Health Conference**, Ministry of Health Documentation Center,
1987.

COSTA, P. P. From projects to public policy: reconstructing the history of
permanent health education. Rio de Janeiro: **FIOCRUZ**, 2006.

Available at: Available at:< http://www.arca.fiocruz.br/handle/icict/5260>.
Accessed on: July 3, 2017.

D'AVILA, L. S. et al. Adherence to the Permanent Education Program for
Family Doctors in a State in the Southeast Region of Brazil. **Science &**

saùde coletiva [online], v. 19, n. 2, p. 401-416, 2014. Available at:
<http://www.redalyc.org/articulo.oa?id=63030092009>. Accessed on: July 3,
2017.

DIAS, H. S.; LIMA, L. D.; TEIXEIRA, M. A trajectória da política nacional de
reorientação da formação profissional em saù no SUS. **Ciência & saùde
coletiva** [online], vol. 18, n. 6, p. 1613-24, 2013. Disponivel em:
<http://dx.doi.org/10.1590/S1413-81232013000600013. Accessed on: July 3,
2017.

DONABEDIAN, A. The seven pillars of quality. **Archives of Pathology &
Laboratory Medicine**. Chicago, v. 114, n. 11, p. 1115-1118, nov. 1990.
Available at: Accessed on: July 3, 2017.

FARAH, B. F. In-service education, continuing education, permanent health
education: synonyms or different concepts? **Revista APS** [serial on the
Internet], July/December 2003. Available at:
<http://www.ufjf.br/nates/files/2009/12/Tribuna.pdf>. Accessed on: July 3,
2017.

FERRARI, R. A. P.; THOMSON, Z.; MELCHIOR, R. Family health strategy:

profile of doctors and nurses, Londrina, Paranâ. **Semina: Biological and Health Sciences**. Londrina, v. 26, n. 2, p.101-108, jul./dez. 2005. Available at: <http//dx.doi.org/10.5433/1679-0367.2005v26n2p101> Accessed on: July 3, 2017.

FERRAZ, F. Permanent health education policies and programs in Brazil: an integrative literature review. **Health & Social Transformation** [electronic version]. Federal University of Santa Catarina, v. 3, n. 2, p. 113-128, 2012. Available at: <http://incubadora.periodicos.ufsc.br/index.php/saudeetransformacao/article/view/1488>. Accessed on: July 3, 2017.

FIGUEIREDO, A. M. **Evaluation of primary health care: analysis of agreement between the AMQ and PCATool instruments in the municipality of Curitiba, Paranâ**. Porto Alegre: Biblioteca FAMED/ HCPA, 2011. Disponivel em:http://www.bibliotecadigital.ufrgs.br/da.php?nrb=000785447&loc=2011&l=17f62592879de47f. Accessed on: June 24, 2014.

FRACOLLI L. A. et al. Primary Health Care evaluation tools: literature review and meta-synthesis. **Ciênc. Saùde Coletiva** [Internet], v. 19, n. 12, p. 4851-4860, 2014. Available at: http://www.scielo.br/scielo.php?script=sci_arttext&pid=S1413-81232014001204851&lng=en. http://dx.doi.org/10.1590/1413-812320141912.00572014. Accessed on: July 3, 2017.

GENEAU, R. et al. Primary care practice a la carte among GPs: using organizational diversity to increase job satisfaction. **BMC Family Practice**, v. 24, n. 2, p. 138-44, 2007. Available at: <https://www.ncbi.nlm.nih.gov/pmc/articles/PMC5020554/>. Accessed on: July 3, 2017.

GIL, C. R. R. Atençâo primària, atençâo bàsica e saùde da familia: synergies and singularities of the Brazilian context. **Cadernos de Saùde Pùblica** [online], v. 22, n. 6, p. 1171-1181, 2006. Disponivel em:< http://dx.doi.org/10.1590/S0102-311X2006000600006>. Accessed on: 03 Jul. 2017.

GOMES, A. P. et al. Primary health care and medical training: between episteme and praxis. **Revista Brasileira de Educaçâo Mèdica**, v. 36 n. 4, p. 541-549, 2012. Available at:< http://dx.doi.org/10.1590/S0100-55022012000600014>. Accessed on: July 3, 2017.

GONZALEZ, A. D.; ALMEIDA, M. J. de. Movements of change in health training: from community medicine to curriculum guidelines.

Physis - Revista de Saùde Coletiva, Rio de Janeiro, v. 20, n. 2, p. 551-570, 2010. Available at:< http://dx.doi.org/10.1590/S0103- 73312010000200012. >. Accessed on: July 3, 2017.

HARZHEIM, E. et al. Validation of the primary health care instrument: PCATool-Brazil adults. **Revista Brasileira de Medicina de Familia e Comunidade**, Rio de Janeiro, v. 8, n. 29, p. 274-284, Oct/Dec. 2013.

Available at:< http://dx.doi.org/10.5712/rbmfc8(29)829>. Accessed on: July 3, 2017.

HAUSER L. et al. Translation, adaptation, validity and reliability measures of the Primary Health Care Assessment Tool (PCATool) in Brazil: health professionals version. **Revista Brasileira de Medicina de Familia e Comunidade**, Rio de Janeiro, v. 8, n. 29, p. 244-255, Oct/Dec.

2013. Available at:< http://dx.doi.org/10.5712/rbmfc8(29)821>. Accessed on: July 3, 2017.

HULLEY, S.B. et al. **Designing Clinical Research**. 2. ed. Philadelphia: Lippincott Williams & Wilkins, 2001.

IBGE. Brazilian Institute of Geography and Statistics. **Yearbook 2012**.

Available at: http://www.goiania.go.gov.br/shtml/seplam/anuario_seplam.pdf>. Accessed on: Aug. 28, 2014.

IBGE. Brazilian Institute of Geography and Statistics. **Estimates of the population of Brazilian municipalities with reference date July 1, 2014** [Nota Tècnica on line]. Available at: http://www.ibge.go.gov.br/home/presidencia/noticias/pdf/analise_estimativas_2014.pdf>. Accessed on: Aug. 28, 2014.

JESUS, M. C. P. et al. Continuing education in nursing in a university hospital. **Revista da Escola de Enfermagem da USP**, Sâo Paulo, v. 45, n. 5, p. 1229-1236, Oct. 2011. Available at: <http://www.ee.usp.br/reeusp/upload/pdf/742.pdf>. Accessed on: July 3, 2017.

KISIL M., CHAVES M. **Programa UNI:** uma nova iniciativa na educação dos profissionais de saúde. Battle Creek: W. K. Kellogg Foundation, 1994.

KOLLING, J. H. G. **Orientation to Primary Health Care in Family Health Teams in the municipalities of the Telessaùde RS project: a baseline study**. Porto Alegre: Biblioteca FAMED/ HCPA, 2008. Disponivel em:http://www.bibliotecadigital.ufrgs.br/da.php?nrb=000785447&loc=2011&l= 17f62592879de47f. Accessed on: June 24, 2014.

LEÂO, C. D. A.; CALDEIRA, A. P. Evaluation of the association between qualification of doctors and nurses in primary health care and quality of care. **Ciência & Saùde Coletiva** [online], v. 16, n. 11, p. 4415-4423, 2011. Available at:< http://dx.doi.org/10.1590/S1413- 81232011001200014>. Accessed on: July 3, 2017.

LEÂO, C. D.; CALDEIRA, A. P.; DE OLIVEIRA, M. M. C. Attributes of primary care in child health care: evaluation of caregivers.

Brazilian Journal of Maternal and Child Health. Recife, v. 11, p. 323-34, jul/set. 2011. Available at:< http://dx.doi.org/10.1590/S1519- 38292011000300013>. Accessed on: July 3, 2017.

LUZ, F. M. da. **Permanent Education in Health (EPS): A strategy that enables transformations in the work process**. Varginha: NESCON/ Faculdade de Medicina/ UFMG, 2010. Available at: https://www.nescon.medicina.ufmg.br/biblioteca/registro/Educacao_Permane nte_em_Saude__EPS___uma_estrategia_que_possibilita_transformacoes_n o_processo_de_trabalho/70. Accessed on: August 30, 2014.

MACHADO, J. L. M.; CALDAS JR, A. L.; BORTONCELLO, N. M. F. A new initiative in the training of health professionals. **Interface (Botucatu)**, Botucatu , v. 1, n. 1, p. 147-156, Aug. 1997 . Available at: <http://www.scielo.br/scielo.php?script=sci_arttext&pid=S1414- 32831997000200011&lng=en&nrm=iso>. Accessed on July 5, 2017.

MACHADO, M. H. et al. **Perfil dos Médicos e Enfermeiros do Programa de Saùde da Familia**. 1. ed. Brasilia: Ministério da Saùde, 2000. v. 6. 592p.

MACIEL, E. L. N. et al. Evaluation of the graduates of the Family Health specialization course in Espirito Santo, Brazil. **Ciênc. Saùde coletiva** [online], v.15, n. 4, p. 2021-2028, 2010. Available at: <http://www.redalyc.org/articulo.oa?id=63018747016>. Accessed on: July 3, 2017.

MACINKO, J. et al. Going to scale with community based primary care an analysis of the family health program and infant mortality in Brazil, 19992004. **Social Science & Medicine**, v. 65, p. 2070-2080, 2007. Available at: < https://doi.org/10.1016/j.socscimed.2007.06.028>. Accessed on: July 3, 2017.

MACINKO, J.; ALMEIDA, C.; SA, P. A rapid assessment methodology for the evaluation of primary care organization and performance in Brazil. **Health Policy and Planning** [Oxford Journals], v. 22, p. 167-177, 2007. Available at: < https://www.ncbi.nlm.nih.gov/pubmed/17400576 >. Accessed on: July 3, 2017.

MACINKO, J.; GUANAIS, F. C.; SOUZA, M. F. M. Evaluation of the impact of the Family Health Program on infant mortality in Brazil: 1990-2002. **Journal of Epidemiology & Community Health**, London, v. 60, n. 1, p. 13-19, 2006. Available at: < https://www.ncbi.nlm.nih.gov/pmc/articles/PMC2465542/ >. Accessed on: July 3, 2017.

MINAYO, M. C. S. Pôs-graduaçâo em Saùde Coletiva de 1997 a 2007: desafios, avanços e tendências. **Ciência & Saùde Coletiva**, Rio de Janeiro, v.15 n. 4, p. 1897-1907, 2010. Available at:

<http://dx.doi.org/10.1590/S1413-81232010011700001>. Accessed on: July 3, 2017.

NASCIMENTO, A. C. **Attributes of Primary Care in Oral Health: an evaluation using the Primary Care Assessment Tool**. Curitiba: PUC/PR, 2011. Available at:

<http://www.biblioteca.pucpr.br/tede/tde_busca/arquivo.php?codArquivo=207 6>. Accessed on: June 24, 2014.

NEGRI, B. **Human Resources in Health. Politics, Development and the Labor Market.** Campinas: Unicamp, 2002. 431 p.

OLIVEIRA, E. B. et al. Evaluation of the quality of care for the elderly in public primary health care services in Porto Alegre, Brazil. **Revista Brasileira de Medicina de Familia e Comunidade**, Rio de Janeiro, v. 8, n. 29, p. 264-73, Oct/Dec. 2013. Available at: <http://hdl.handle.net/10183/140034>. Accessed on: July 3, 2017.

OLIVEIRA, F. M. C. S. N. et al. Continuing education and quality of health care: meaningful learning in nursing work. **Aquichan**, Bogotà, v. 11, n. 1, apr. 2011. Available at:< http://www.redalyc.org/html/741/74118880005/>. Accessed on: July 3, 2017.

Oliveira, M. P. R. et al. Training and Qualification of Health Professionals: Factors Associated with the Quality of Primary Care. **Revista Brasileira de Educaçâo Mèdica.** n. 40 v. 4, p. 547-559, 2016. Disponivel em:

http://dx.doi.org/10.1590/1981-52712015v40n4e02492014. Accessed on: July 3, 2017.

PAHO, CONASS. **The implementation of the chronic conditions care model in Curitiba.** Constitution of the Federative Republic of Brazil: results of the innovation laboratory on care for chronic conditions in primary health care. Brasilia: Pan American Health Organization, National Council of Health Secretaries, 2013.

WORLD HEALTH ORGANIZATION. **Declaration of Alma Ata**. Kazajstàn: WHO; 1978.

PAIM, J. et al. The Brazilian health system: history, advances and challenges. **The Lancet** [online], London, p. 11-31, May 2011. Available at:< http://www.cpgss.pucgoias.edu.br/ArquivosUpload/31/file/O%20SISTEMA%2 0DE%20SAUDE%20BRASILEIRO.pdf >. Accessed on: July 3, 2017.

PEDUZZI, M. et al. Educational activities of workers in primary care: conceptions of permanent education and continuing education in health present in the daily life of Basic Health Units in São Paulo. **Interface (Botucatu)**, Botucatu, v. 13, n. 30, sep. 2009. Disponivel em:< http://dx.doi.org/10.1590/S1414-32832009000300011>. Accessed on: July 3, 2017.

RIBEIRO, F. A. **Atençâo Primària (APS) e sistema de saù no Brasil: uma perspectiva histórica**. Sâo Paulo: Faculty of Medicine/ USP, 2007. Available at: http://www.teses.usp.br/teses/disponiveis/5/5137/tde- 24102007-084507/en-br.php. Accessed on: Aug. 30, 2014.

ROCHA, B. S. **Nurses from the Family Health Program - Team Coordinators: professional, technical and interpersonal profile.**

Goiânia: Faculty of Nursing/UFG, 2008. Available at: http://repositorio.bc.ufg.br/tede/handle/tde/746. Accessed on: Aug. 30, 2014.

RONCALLI, A; LIMA, K. Impacto do PSF sobre indicadores de saù da criança em municipios de grande porte do Nordeste do Brasil. **Ciência & Saùde Coletiva**, v. 11, p. 713-724, 2006. Available at:< https://repositorio.ufrn.br/jspui/handle/123456789/20846 >. Accessed on: July 3, 2017.

SHI, L. Primary care, specialty care and life chances. **International Journal of Health Services**, v. 24, n. 3, p. 431-458, 1994. Available at: <https://www.ncbi.nlm.nih.gov/pubmed/7928012>. Accessed on: July 3, 2017.

STARFIELD, B. **Primary care: balancing health needs, services and technology**. Brasilia: UNESCO, MS, 2002. 726p.

TESSER, C. D. et al. Family Health Strategy and social reality analysis: subsidies for health promotion and continuing education policies. **Ciência & saùde coletiva** [online], v. 16, n. 11, p. 4295-4306, 2011. Available at:< http://dx.doi.org/10.1590/S1413- 81232011001200002>. Accessed on: July 3, 2017.

TOMASI, E. et al. Socio-demographic and epidemiological profile of primary health care workers in the South and Northeast regions of Brazil. **Cadernos de Saùde Pùblica**, Rio de Janeiro, n. 24, p. 193-201,2008. Available at:< http://dx.doi.org/10.1590/S0102-311X2008001300023 >. Accessed on: July 3, 2017.

VITORIA, A. M., et al. Evaluation of the attributes of primary health care in Chapecó, Brazil. **Revista Brasileira de Medicina de Familia e Comunidade**, Rio de Janeiro, v. 8, n. 29, p. 285-293, Oct/Dec. 2013.

Available at: <http://dx.doi.org/10.5712/rbmfc8(29)832>. Accessed on: July 3, 2017.

ZILS, A. M. et al. Satisfaction of users of the Primary Care network in Porto Alegre. **Revista Brasileira de Medicina de Familia e Comunidade**, Rio de Janeiro, v. 4, n. 16, p. 270-276, jan/mar. 2009. Available at: <http://dx.doi.org/10.5712/rbmfc4(16)233>. Accessed on: July 3, 2017.

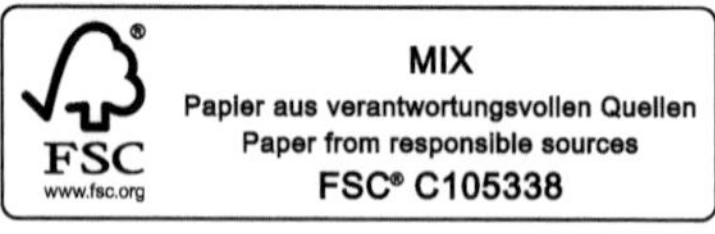

MIX
Papier aus verantwortungsvollen Quellen
Paper from responsible sources
FSC® C105338
FSC
www.fsc.org